Public Health and Society

Public Health and Society

John Costello and Monica Haggart

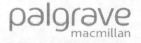

First published 2003 by
PALGRAVE MACMILLAN
Houndmills, Basingstoke, Hampshire RG21 6XS and
175 Fifth Avenue, New York, N.Y. 10010
Companies and representatives throughout the world

PALGRAVE MACMILLAN is the global academic imprint of the Palgrave
Macmillan division of St. Martin's Press, LLC and of Palgrave Macmillan Ltd.
Macmillan® is a registered trademark in the United States, United Kingdom
and other countries. Palgrave is a registered trademark in the European
Union and other countries.

ISBN 0–333–97173–6 paperback

This book is printed on paper suitable for recycling and made from fully
managed and sustained forest sources.

A catalogue record for this book is available from the British Library.

10   9   8   7   6   5   4   3   2   1
12   11   10   09   08   07   06   05   04   03

Printed and bound in Great Britain by
Creative Print and Design (Wales), Ebbw Vale

Contents

Contents

List of Figures and Tables

Foreword

In Chapter 1 of this book the age-old question of the definition of public health is quite properly comprehensively reviewed. I have always liked the definition favoured by Alwyn Smith – that epidemiology is the *study* of the health of human communities and public health is the *practice* of *improving* the health of human communities. This begs of course the definition of 'health' and 'community'.

There is another debate that flows from this definition – is epidemiology a biological science or a social science, and is public health a branch of the health professions or a branch of social administration? This is a debate which will run endlessly because important issues of status, identity and territory rest on it. And yet it is a nonsense for the only possible answer to each question is 'Both'.

A public health professional must understand the hard statistical and biological evidence of what it is that disturbs health and that causes death, disability, illness and distress in human beings. How else can they set their agenda? But unless that is linked to an understanding of the behaviours, cultures, norms, economics and politics that shape the social and physical environment in which the determinants of health are rooted, epidemiology will, as Alwyn Smith has commented, forever remain a mass of surgically clean data untouched by human thought, and public health practice will be a process of analysis not change. Neither Disraeli nor Marx are fashionable these days but Marx's comments that the aim is 'to change society not to understand it', and that 'human beings are the masters of their own destiny but not in the circumstances of their own choosing' are eminently valid in public health practice, as is Disraeli's rallying cry that 'the health of the people is the first concern of Government'. Indeed if we counterpose Disraeli's statement with Lenin's comment that 'the health of the people is the concern of the people themselves' we can recognise a key tension in public health practice, with the strange paradox that the words of Lenin would fit best in the mouths of Conservative Governments whereas it seems to be Labour Governments that have heard the voice of Disraeli.

It is timely therefore for John Costello and Monica Haggart to attempt a review of the relations of public health and society. It is an ambitious task and one in which no contribution can be definitive. But I believe that they have produced a significant contribution to the evolution of ideas.

This book is not the answer to the questions it poses – it will have succeeded if it causes public health practitioners to think about them.

Stephen J. Watkins
Director of Public Health for Stockport

Preface

This book is intended for practitioners working in community health settings and student nurses undertaking a community placement. Its primary focus is public health using sociological theory to develop ideas about health and illness across a broad spectrum of society. The purpose of the book is to provide those working in public health roles and their students with a text which gives an overview of health, need and service provision. Each of the chapters sets out to demonstrate the link between health care provision and the social structures that underpin the services to a range of people, including families and individuals. The three main themes of the book are power, control and professionalisation and each part of the book reflects the three themes which are dealt with in more detail within specific chapters. The book reviews historical developments in public health provision, and takes a critical look at the way in which health need is intrinsically linked with social and political change. The book is organised into three parts, each of which interrelate.

Part I   Public Health and Nursing: Origins and Development

The first three chapters of the book trace the historical, social and political issues which impinge on the provision of public health and use sociological theory and policy to highlight how public health arose historically from a synthesis of ideas about health and illness as well as a need for political change to improve individual and community health. Chapter 1 considers the origins and direction of traditional and what is called 'new' public health and examines traditional and contemporary debates on the topic. Chapter 2 looks at the individual and social factors which impinge on health and how individuals can often feel disempowered, when trying to become and stay healthy, by the actions of professionals who are responsible for promoting health. Chapter 3 examines the relationship between social and health inequalities and takes a critical look at health care in Victorian England, examining how public health changes took place as a result of social change and medical innovation. It then focuses on the implications of the Black report and beyond in terms of the impact that health reforms have on changing the underlying causes of disease and illness.

Part II Public Health and Control: Social Responsibility for the Promotion of Health

Part II of the book (Chapters 4, 5 and 6) examines the need for public health services and their utilisation by vulnerable groups, including those from diverse communities (Chapter 4). Chapter 4 looks at the experiences of ethnic minority groups in Britain and focuses on the Chinese community as an illustration of how traditional values and beliefs about health can coexist within the ideology of Western medicine. Chapter 5 looks at vulnerable social groups and, using case study material, illustrates how vulnerability can be created by social forces that seek to marginalise certain members of society. The chapter examines the way in which powerful institutions influence the vulnerability of some people and keeps them out of the mainstream of society. Chapter 6 examines the way media constructions of health provision influence our thinking about health and offers a critique of the way in which health promotion is manipulated by powerful media forces to conjurer up a false, and sometimes humorous, way of considering health in contemporary society.

Part III Measuring and Managing Public Health: Current and Future Perspectives

Chapters 7, 8 and 9 are designed to enable the reader to look at the way public health is currently assessed and measured in contemporary society and the way government responses shape the way social problems are dealt with. Chapter 7 illustrates the social diversity of need as well as the problems associated with providing public health services to those who are often at the periphery of society and whose needs are often the most difficult to meet. Chapter 8 focuses on social exclusion and the work of the Government's Social Exclusion Units (SEUs), critically examining political responses to public health, and considering how far political change has influenced the fundamental problem of social inequality. Individual case studies highlight different social issues and are used to illustrate the processes involved in social exclusion. The final chapter looks at the future of public health and the need for a professional response to assess the role of public health nursing in the provision of a clear framework for the developing public health services.

Throughout the book a number of public health issues are addressed using theoretical and practical examples based on case studies and research evidence. The book is not intended as a polemic text; rather, it is the authors' intention to provide the reader with a broad overview that critically examines the provision of health services and provides ideas about how to develop and improve the practical care that is the essence of public health.

We hope that community health practitioners and their students find the book stimulating and useful to their practice as well as valuable for developing future studies into health care.

John Costello and Monica Haggart
September 2002

Acknowledgements

This book has had a long gestation and we have been given advice, suggestions, and helpful comments from numerous sources. In particular we would like to acknowledge the support and advice provided by our colleagues in professional practice and to thank them for helping to represent and hopefully 'make real' much of the writing.

We would also like to acknowledge the hard work and patience of the chapter contributors who have put a great deal of effort into the compilation of this work. Numerous others have been sources of inspiration notably Joanne Kerr and Jeff Edwards.

In particular, we would like to acknowledge the support from our families for their encouragement, patience and passing on of many messages. A special acknowledgement goes to John Rees, for his tireless help with reading and re-reading many of the chapters. Many thanks also to the team at Palgrave Macmillan, particularly Jon Reed and Magenta Lampson for their support throughout the writing of this book.

Notes on the Contributors

Ross Brocklehurst is a nursing lecturer (teaching) and Programme Leader at the University of Manchester School of Nursing, Midwifery and Health Visiting.

John Costello is a lecturer in nursing and research fellow at the University of Manchester School of Nursing, Midwifery and Health Visiting.

Monica Haggart is a health visiting lecturer (teaching) at the University of Manchester School of Nursing, Midwifery and Health Visiting and leads the community specialist practitioner course.

Maria Horne is a health visiting lecturer (teaching) at the University of Manchester School of Nursing, Midwifery and Health Visiting.

Ron Iphofen is a senior lecturer in sociology of health at the school of Nursing, Midwifery and Health Studies, University of Wales, Bangor.

Martin King is a senior lecturer in sociology in the Department of Health Care Studies, Manchester Metropolitan University, Faculty of Health and Applied Community Studies.

Joel Richman, is a professor Emeritus of anthropology at Manchester Metropolitan University.

Maryam Spanswick is a district nurse working in Plant Hill Clinic, Blackley, North Manchester.

Louise Wong is a mental health development worker at the Women's Chinese Society in Manchester.

Part I

Public Health and Nursing: Origins and Development

1

Holding Public Health Up for Inspection

JOEL RICHMAN

The key points discussed in this chapter include:

- public health definitions: the political and social significance of public health in contemporary society

- key historical public health changes that have influenced the development of public health in the UK

- the link between industrialisation and the development of the 'new public health' in the twentieth century.

Introduction

The purpose of this chapter is to consider some of the key definitions of public health, highlighting its importance in terms of its analytical and moral status. In doing this the chapter will develop an historical and cross-cultural perspective on public health, noting the diffusion of public health with colonisation (an 'early stage' of globalisation). Public health is a multiplex concept consisting of a wide range of interpretations, social, political and economic, with many lay and professional practices, values and ideas embedded within it. From a sociological point of view, consideration is made of the various debates about the 'new' public health and especially whether it constitutes a new social movement with a modern health agenda. This necessitates the provision of an outline of some of the discussions about public health within current health delivery. The chapter concludes with a consideration of lay beliefs and their importance in defining ideas about health, as well as a look forward to some of the underpinning issues associated with public health which will hopefully sensitise the reader to their more substantial unfolding in later chapters.

Differing Perspectives on Public Health

Public health has been variously described as 'old' and 'new'. Ashton and Seymour (1988) locate the 'old' within the excesses of industrialisation in Europe and North America; rapid urbanisation, overcrowding and squalor; one-third of the population of Manchester (1821) living in cellars (see Engels, 1982). Contagious diseases were rampant: smallpox, cholera, tuberculosis and measles. Public health based on environmental interventions was then called the 'Sanitary Movement', spearheaded by medical officers of health armed with National Public Health Acts, for example 1848 and 1875. The 'New Public Health' (often assumed to originate from the report of Lalonde, Canadian Minister of Health, 'New Perspective on the Health of Canadians', 1974) transforms the environment into the social and psychological, with the promotion of healthy life-styles, individual responsibility and risk reduction.

There are numerous perspectives that may be developed on public health, although a focus will be placed on three key approaches that encapsulate much of the debate taking place in the current and last century. First is the belief that we, as consumers, have taken responsibility and control of our own health. This belief incorporates the idea that public health has professional and lay dimensions. The latter focuses on the idea that we, as consumers, are responsible for our own health and historically demonstrates how there has been a shift in power between the professionals and the consumer. It may be argued we are now advised and taught by the professional experts about what we need to do in order to stay healthy (Illich, 1976). Second, and in a related way, it is clear that power relations between the health professional and the client have changed and we no longer need feel that we are dependent on the experts. Third, the notion of health being available from within large institutions such as hospitals is changing and, although we see health care becoming more available, the idea of institutional care is an important part of our awareness of public health (Acheson, 1988).

Public health practitioners (as discussed by Haggart in Chapter 9), recognise that most illness episodes are treated by self-medication with a limited contribution made by health professionals. Diet and exercise are promoted for reducing the demands on the medical hegemony. In Woody Allen's quip, 'you eat brown rice and live forever', we see evidence of the idea that becoming healthy is one issue but staying healthy and being healthy are matters for individual compulsion. Illich (1976) further argued that people should stop being addicted to medicine, that is, having cultural iatrogenesis. Medicine, Illich argues, has mystified everyday life, making us a passive commodity of its production. In order to take responsibility for our own health we need to become more active in challenging medical beliefs but at the same time develop a more positive orientation and take responsibility for maintaining an optimum level of health. This works well if you are in reasonably good health to begin with and there are no major social issues impinging on your life chances such as poverty or unemployment affecting your health.

The role of the patient has changed and increasingly we are exposed to the idea that we are less dependent on the professional and in the process have become more liberated health consumers. This, as King points out in Chapter 6, has been partly due to the influence of the media in drawing our attention to healthy images and the need for us to develop and become better role models for our children. Does the image of the 'couch potato' conjure up a negative enough image to make us want to start that diet right away? Historically, there has been a shift in power so that we now may be seen as agents of our own health futures. At the same time, however, we are seeing increasing evidence of the non-compliant patient (refuses to obey doctor's orders) becoming a health negotiator, wanting to know why we take the medication, for how long and what the side effects will do.

The third perspective being drawn upon is the idea that health delivery is 'out there' and health is institutionally based. This is an issue discussed in more detail by Haggart in Chapter 9. Historically, the Ancient Greeks, for example, regarded health as part of the cultural component of society and fully visible. Today there are debates as to how far medical control, institutionally based, with its high technological intervention, should contribute to public health. Specifically, feminists, citing the over-use of Caesarian sections, have argued that birth is too high tech. Foetal monitoring is only needed in $2:3,000$ cases. The Caesarean section rate of 25 per cent has doubled in the last twenty years (the UK having the highest rate in Europe, Richman, 1987). WHO guidance suggests that Caesareans in developed countries should be no more than 10 per cent. The shortage of midwives has been one of the thrusts behind the increase in hospital Caesarean birth and minimal domiciliary delivery.

What is Public Health?

For many, public health is 'taken for granted' with no need for definition. Le Fanu's (1999) prize-winning *Rise and Fall of Modern Medicine* does not index 'public health'. Instead, a chapter titled 'Seduced by Social Theory' notes public health targets and is critical of the changing and contradictory health advice provided by certain food manufacturers as 'going beyond common knowledge' (p. 314) and causing illnesses. Porter's (1997) *magnum opus*, a history of medicine from 'antiquity' to the present does index public health's diverse activities but still does not offer a working definition. Contemporary policy documents such as *The NHS Plan* (DoH, 2000), the template of government policy, sets out a myriad health targets but also omits a public health definition. None of its sections discusses public health. Of the 134 contributors to the plan (Modernisation Action Team Members), only two have the title 'public health' attached to them. Despite this, we are informed by Griffiths and Hunter (1999) that public health has become more fashionable since Labour came to power in 1997 and the appointment of the first Minister for Public Health.

Earlier writers, for example, Brockington (1960) gave more extensive definitions of public health:

> The application of hygiene, the science which seeks to preserve health to the body corporate, the community. All knowledge which can help to maintain its health, social, scientific and medical, comes within its purview; medicine plays a predominant but not exclusive role.

It is noteworthy how the nineteenth-century residuality of public health lingered and that medical knowledge, although differently systematised, was still regarded as amicable towards the public health enterprise. This definition relied heavily upon the WHO (1952) extensive framework for public health, a global birthright of health and longevity:

> The science and art of preventing disease … promoting health and efficiency through organised community efforts for the sanitation of the environment, control of communicable infections and the education of the individual in personal hygiene, the organisation of the medical and nursing services for early diagnosis and preventive treatment of disease and development of social machinery to ensure for every individual a standard of living adequate for the maintenance of health.

The WHO promotes public health as a fully integrated system, with 'community' as a core unit of social action, but fails to explicate *types* of political, power relationships necessary for tranformatory health relations.

The Meaning of Public Health

It would appear that definitions of public health are of limited substance. There is no attempt to define key components, for example, 'community' and 'public', which appear to be used synonymously. Hillery (1995) identified 94 definitions of community; all they had in common was some agreement that it involved people! There are examples of how such connections have been made in the past, such as the de-institutionalisation of psychiatric hospitals that was similarly predicated on the belief that 'community' was a term which exuded warmth and emotional well-being (Tonnies, 1957). The chameleon of community soon merges with another taken-for-granted, 'environment', and more recently the politically engineered Primary Care Trusts. However, the Jakarta Declaration (1999) did add the refinement that both the public and private sectors should promote health and restrict harmful substances like weapons. To overcome the above difficulties some writers resort to a trait (activity) representation of public health, which is continuously multiplying to now include resistance to antibiotics and fluoridation (once heavily promoted by the dental profession). The latter is now considered an infringement of personal rights. Griffiths and Hunter (1991:1) succinctly sum up our position: 'One of the problems with public health is that it can be everything – the air, the food or water, health behaviours, health sciences.'

The meanings behind public health are often not made clear. In particular, the varied perceptions of 'social health problem' are not explicated, especially when a global perspective is adopted which increasingly happens when using comparative data on health (see Costello *et al.*, Chapter 4 re globalisation issues). Looking at the differing meanings of public health causes the reader to consider to what extent is the reality of public health separate from the rhetoric about health care in general. To develop a wider perspective, then, a closer look at different perceptions of public health is required.

Perceptions of Public Health

For public health to be regarded as 'totemic', a guide to our sense, it is better to explicate the three categories of thought enmeshed in public health.

First, public health is a *moral category*. To be healthy implies to be in harmony; how and with what raises huge epistemological questions of an essentially philosophical hue requiring cross-cultural reference. Illness is a deviation from accepted standards of well-being. Plato argued, for example, that on balance a healthy life would be more pleasurable. Public health takes this stance, implying it is a moral duty to maintain good health by adopting appropriate practices. Burls (2000:148) comments: 'Many public health practitioners take it for granted that, since their role is to work on behalf of populations to produce *maximum* health gain, utilitarian principles provide the fundamental ethical framework to guide their decisions' (our emphasis). Whether we like it or not we have a duty to have longevity.

Public health is also a *prescriptive category*. leading from the above, public health, like the Talmud or the Koran, injects a sense of religiosity – to do some things and avoid others. It creates new taboos and duties. We have to work at being healthy, following the Protestant Work Ethic – as in the gym, with 'no pain, no gain' as a new mantra. The public health gaze defines the world into opposites based on risk–danger/safety. Before we put a supermarket product in our basket it must be critically scrutinised for threatening additives. The risk–danger factor is under constant revision – it's our duty to educate ourselves about changes (margarine is now a risk product for example). It's now a duty to participate publicly – democracy in health decisions. The NHS Plan was not only hinged to a patient-centred health service but also has proposals to increase public involvement.

Finally public health is an *analytical category*. Through public health methodologies we are able to reach a greater 'truth' about our existence by demonstrating that this or that is valid. Public health contains the tools for evaluating the effectiveness of clinical practice and health interventions; cost-effectiveness and prioritisation (rationing of health) are some of the goals of public health. Public health practitioners are now front-line workers who, with their skills, can map out the needs of a local population and, to some extent, guard the perimeter of infection for families. They are also expected to increase the health resources of their patch – how, is by no means clear. It is expected that by contact with public health practitioners some of their skills/knowledge will pass to consumers like a laying on of hands. However, the role of a public health practitioner is variable and open ended, one that has to emerge by praxis. It is for that reason we now go on to locate the changing patterns of public health according to different contexts, to analyse whether there are threads of continuity.

The Origins of Public Health:
Historical Perspectives

Brockington (1960:3) perceptibly noted that public health, in some form, has existed as long as civilisation. 'Inoculation against smallpox was practised in India and in China before the Christian era. Isolation of leprosy was enforced in the Roman Empire, which built leprosaria: the first isolation hospitals ... many religious abstentions concerned food and excretal pollution.' Public health historians differ, however, regarding the societies to be taken as benchmarks. Rosen (1993) considers five critical periods: Greco-Roman; Middle Ages, with the devastating Black Death and related plagues wiping out over 30 per cent of the European population; Age of Absolutism (1500–1750); Age of Enlightenment (the foundation of rationality); and

Age of Industrialisation, from 1830 onwards. Brockington considers 'early public health' up to 1830 and then nineteenth-century and twentieth-century public health.

Classical Greek and Roman

The Romans engineered safe water and sanitary latrines, dating from 3000 BC in Crete. The Romans, especially, created a military medical service; each doctor, given a commissioned rank, looked after five hundred men. Alexander the Great's achievements would have been impossible without his 'field doctors'. The two rival Greek medical traditions based on Cnidos (which stressed the disease and elaborate classification) and Cos (emphasising the patient) were empirically based on observation, removing divine causation. Hippocrates (460–377 BC) in particular argued that epilepsy (sacred disease) had natural causations. In his '*Airs, Waters, Places*' (which can be read as a treatise on public health) he put great emphasis on the environment for well-being. He advised physicians arriving at an unfamiliar town to examine its position in terms of wind and sun. Florence Nightingale was also a great believer in 'invigorating winds/ventilation'. Broadmoor hospital was chosen for these healing qualities. Hippocrates noted that marshy waters gave rise to summer epidemics of dysentery, diarrhoea and malaria. The notion of 'miasmic disorders' lasted until the late nineteenth century.

Medieval and Renaissance Public Health

This was a period when Greek and Arabic medical texts were 'rediscovered'. (In fact, Arabic medicine had kept Greek medical thought alive and translated many texts into Arabic.) For example, Alphanus, a Benedictine monk, voyaged to Constantinople in the eleventh century to acquaint himself with Greek texts. The Salernitan Programme of Health emphasised hygiene, diet and exercise as the basis of good living. Porter (1997:107) refers to it as the 'first home health manual'. The dominance of the Church set a rigid framework for medieval practice. Plagues were caused by divine retribution, or by Jewish unbelievers. Death was a church monopoly. The Church set up a register of approved physicians, usually clerics. Pilgrimages and healing shrines, especially dedicated to saints, were recommended. Epilepsy again became a divine illness. Hospitals expanded to treat returning crusaders. In the thirteenth century the professionalisation of doctors took off (for example, 1367 was the Fellowship of English Surgeons). The north Italian city states, Aragon and Valencia, by 1300 had installed public physicians, later being emulated by the German cities. British cities were slow to adopt this policy. Cities swollen by trading activities initiated public health measures, Bruges being a leader in installing an integrated water and sewage network. To avoid increased pollution, certain tradespeople like slaughterers and dyers were not allowed to dump their waste in public drinking water facilities.

Lepers abounded and were stigmatised; forced into ghettos outside towns, made to comply with distinct 'dress codes' and sounding a bell when people came near. They were subjected to many rites of exclusion; forbidden to marry or to be buried in public cemeteries. Porter (1997:122) estimates that there were 19,000 leprosaria in Europe by 1225. When leprosy died out (no one knows why) the mentally ill, associated with witchcraft, became the new polluting outsiders, often being given to travelling merchants, drowned or locked away.

The largest threat came from periodic plague, often following trade routes from the Levant and China as did the 1347–51 bubonic pandemic. Doctors had no cure. Fires were lit in streets, as the Greeks had done, to disperse the so-called 'contagious miasma'. Commissioners for Public Health, now medical magistrates, with doctors relegated to advisors, were first set up in fifteenth-century Italian city states. Quarantine of people and goods was the only remedy against the plague.

The Golden Age of Public Health

The golden age of public health is regarded by many as the nineteenth and early twentieth century. During this time, many public health measures were fully institutionalised and engrained in reforming Parliamentary Acts. This section will examine the claims that the latter were more instrumental in raising the nation's health than clinical practices *per se*, as suggested by McKeown (1976, 1979) among others. The role of Florence Nightingale, as a leader of this sanitary movement and developer of community nursing, will also be explored. The impact of early globalisation, for example economic competition from Germany and colonial development, is another public health theme on display. The 'Sanitarian Movement' from the 1830s was stimulated by the morbidity and the mortality toll of rapacious industrialisation. Half of Manchester children died before their fifth birthday. A labourer in Liverpool had a life expectancy of 15 years. Factory reforms, for example, were not entirely based on humanitarian/moral grounds. Workers' revolts in Europe had their counterpart in the Chartist's demands. Unemployed workers formed armed gangs. It was important to neutralise growing discontent. (Marx had predicted that the first workers' revolution would be in England because of its advanced stage of industrialisation.)

However as Hamlin (2000) points out, Chadwick, the first leader of the Sanitarians, argued that poor health was not generated by worker poverty (he had devised the New Poor Law 1834, which forbade relief to the unemployed). Chadwick believed that the free market was God's natural gift. He singled out adequate sewage disposal and clean drinking water as the basis of good health (an old idea). Infections like cholera and fevers were due to miasma, toxic air from rotting debris. Miasma, a foul smelling vapour was the dominant illness metaphor before 1860. Sontag (1979) showed how some illnesses, incompletely understood at the time, like TB, came to dominate cultural understandings. Even the rich with good drains and sound body constitution were not immune from miasmatic illness (see Brocklehurst and Costello, Chapter 3 for further discussion). Its 'randomness' was especially linked to chaotic moral standards and rioting by the masses. It was believed that household overcrowding also precipitated mass incest. Miasma also became a metaphor for progress, Chadwick believed that the drains would not only take the filth away, but it could be transformed into fertiliser to increase food production for the expanding towns.

Chadwick's Public Health Act of 1848 created general boards of health, the first in London; they were set up where 10 per cent of the residents petitioned or where the death rate was above 23 per 1,000. Their medical officers were to remove the 'causes' of disease. The first International Public Health Conference 1851 met in Paris with 12 nations debating for six months. Sardinia, Portugal and Russia, for example, promoted increased use of quarantine. England and France subscribed to the miasmic theory. By 1900 ten international conferences had met, and were especially concerned with the spread of cholera.

Florence Nightingale and Public Health

Small (1998) discussed how Florence Nightingale, usually considered a founder of hospital nursing, was a convert to public health care. From her base at Scutari, in the Crimea, Nightingale attempted to improve conditions for soldiers affected more by the lack of hygiene than the conflict on the battlefield. She decided that it was necessary to focus on public health issues in an attempt to provide a more healthy environment. Despite her attempts to improve conditions, between 1854–55 ten times more soldiers died from illness (typhoid, dysentery and cholera) than from battle injuries. Besides learning four languages she was a very competent social statistician, being conversant with the work of Alphonse Quetelet (1796–1874) the Belgian social scientist whose statistical findings Comte, a sociological founder of positivism, incorporated in his technique

'Social Physics' and applied to mortality statistics and crime, discovering regularities (for example, crime was lower in countries of high education). Despite Nightingale's breakdown in 1857 (Small suggests guilt from the high mortality at Scutari) she statistically analysed 'her' failures, for example why soldiers amputated in the field mostly recovered but those in hospital did not. With the help of Dr William Farr, Superintendent of the Statistical Department of Registrar-Generals Office, she produced a confidential report on medical failings during the Crimean War. Farr had studied hygiene in the Paris Medical School, but no English equivalent would allow him to teach it; the medical establishment felt threatened by the subject. He questioned the fashionable miasma theory and attacked the doctors in his first report (1839) for being complacent about the infant mortality of 270 per 1,000. In his book *Philosophy of Health* (Farr, 1836), Farr argues that women were the 'original' health teachers and must become nurses.

Nightingale bombarded the Crimean inquiry with statistics: our mortality from diseases of the stomach and bowels at Scutari was 23.6 per cent, in the Crimea 18.3 per cent (Small, 1998:92). Nightingale later refined 'hygiene' to distinguish between personal (clothing and diets) and building hygiene. She argued that doctors were the wrong people to be in charge of 'building hygiene'. Nightingale was an astute politician, using friends in high places to get over her views based on statistical evidence. She replaced Chadwick as the opinion leader of 'public health'. Chadwick had made many enemies and was contemptible of those not sharing his views, attacking the Government for not supplying adequate funds for sewers. He wanted new taxes for these enterprises and for the middle-class electorate to pay more.

Nightingale's *Notes on Nursing* (1860) elevated 'household hygiene', for example, lack of 'white washing', ventilation, random diets all being the major health hazards. She believed that statistical findings, as nature's laws, should guide public health policy. She was deeply religious (not in a fundamentalist way), having claimed to have visions of God in early life. Florence Nightingale also took a great interest in India, noting that the creation of its own public health department was a noble task, creating India anew by introducing a higher civilisation.

Modern nursing was not only for healing the sick, but also for health promotion. Dossey (2000) claims that Nightingale's public health (care) work was a holistic extension of nursing. She criticised doctors for their excess power but was in favour of compulsory smallpox vaccination, which many anti-medical supporters were not. Idealistically, she looked forward to the abolition of all hospitals. She was opposed to women becoming doctors and also to the registration of nurses. Nightingale had studied nursing as practised by the Augustinians at Kaiserworth and found the 'spirit' more essential to nursing. She regarded nurses more as health missionaries.

The International Dimension of Public Health

The international dimension of public health became more important towards the end of the nineteenth century. (The 1897 International Conference was concerned primarily with the spread of plague by Mecca pilgrims.) Fears had arisen that Britain was experiencing 'national degeneracy'. Economic superiority was challenged by the USA and German competition, the Boer War produced evidence of the unfitness of recruits. The 'dangerous classes' were aptly named: considered the major source of disease, not institutionalised into schools or work, they could be the instant street source of political discontent and their aggressive street behaviour hassled the middle classes, whose birth rate began falling in 1870. The Eugenic Movement was founded (eugenics was a term coined by Galton) to improve the population stock. It had many left-wing supporters like the Webbs, who had suggested compulsory sterilisation of the unfit. This became policy in Sweden, Germany and elsewhere. The Lunacy Act (1890), supported by notable doctors like Maudsley, classified the mentally impaired into lunatics, imbeciles and idiots; their differing degree of pollution/danger related to their spatial separation, like Indian caste. Maternity and child welfare also improved. The Child Study Movement started in 1896. Milk depots based on the Paris model commenced. The Infant Welfare Movement, initially consultation centres, spawned health visitors. To encourage the registration of births, Huddersfield gave one pound to the mother whose child survived a year. District nursing, the prototype of public health nursing, had commenced in 1859.

The USA, whose industrialisation and 'social evils' commenced later than England's, learned much from its experience. Ward (1972), a sociologist, founded the Henry Street Settlement 1893 for district and school nursing. The USA, similarly feared a decline in 'population quality' with the new immigrants from south Europe who took children's care very seriously. It established the Federal Children's Bureau, in 1908. Public health nursing commenced in the USA in 1887, those supported by private agencies were called 'visiting nurses'. Midwives in England and the USA had to be qualified nurses.

Public Health: Home and Abroad

There was a symbiotic relationship between the development of public health in England and in the Empire. The health of the 'native' was taken to be an indicator of good and bad colonial power, with Belgium as the worst colonists. The Congo was treated as a private hunting reserve of King Leopold. Slaves who escaped from the plantations had their feet cut off. The French general, Lyautey, argued that colonialism had many blemishes but was redeemed by the doctor. Florence Nightingale laid plans for irrigation, sewage works, supported famine relief and low interest for peasants' loans. Some administrators did not believe in distributing food during famines; this would disturb the working of the free market. Nightingale supported Indian independence and in the abolition of the salt tax, which later initiated the Ghandi Nationalist Protest Movement. Some diseases were actually transmitted by colonists with syphilis known as 'Firangi Roga', or European disease.

The health of the English colonists, especially the military, was paramount for natives vastly out numbered them. Parkes, Professor of Military Hygiene, recognised the importance of the soldier's diet, with a balance between fats, carbohydrates and salt, with plenty of fresh fruit. Cattle had to be inspected for anthrax and parasites before being consumed. The Army Sanitary Commission from the 1870s improved the ventilation of the barracks. However, Harrison (1994:70) argues that after the discovery by Robert Koch, 'The bacteriological thesis of disease causation heightened European anxiety about the medical dangers of the Indian people, saturated with infection'.

In 1870 one in twenty soldiers was hospitalised with venereal disease: most officers were unmarried, with prostitution the main sexual release. India's Contagious Disease Act of 1870 was modelled on its British counterpart with the compulsory examination of the suspected prostitutes and medical inspection of the brothels. The British Act only applied to small garrison towns, like Portsmouth, the India regulation to wider populations, like Calcutta. The main concern of the British was famine and the cycle of plague, the latter spread more easily by the extensive railway network. The Plague Commission recommended more 'health officers' to improve death registrations, an early warning system of 'plague'. A major ethical issue was whether vaccination against smallpox (introduced in the 1820s) should be compulsory, the debate mirroring its English counterpart on the freedom of choice. The 'cordon sanitaire' was a major defence against cholera, but this sanitary regulation disturbed pilgrimages. Of greater global concern in contemporary times is the spread of diseases such as TB, once thought to been eradicated. Changing patterns of communicable diseases indicate that certain risk factors have emerged as part of a pattern of globalisation (see Costello *et al.*, Chapter 4). Table 1.1 highlights the impact of selected communicable diseases and the threat they pose to global health as well as the environmental risk.

Table 1.1 Selected communicable diseases posing a global
health and environmental risk

Communicable disease	Selected data

Tuberculosis bacilli	One-third of world's population are carriers
	Kills 3 million people annually
	DOTs cost US $3–5 per healthy year of
	  life and prevents drug resistance which
	  costs up to 100 times more to treat

HIV/AIDS	Infected up to 24 million adults of whom 4 million have died

Viral hepatitis	At least 350 million people are chronic
	  carriers of hepatitis B and 100 million
	  have hepatitis C

Global health

In the late nineteenth century nurses worked in the colonies after their
heroism in the Crimea. The Colonial Nursing Association (1895) sponsored suitable candidates, often those with missionaries and doctors as
relatives. Initially they nursed Europeans, and were subject to strict sexual
regulations keeping them apart from the natives. They were primarily
administrators, running the wards with native nurses (often men) under
training. European styles of care were introduced, relatives being forbidden to cook on the wards for their sick kin.

The colonies, especially Africa, became a 'laboratory' for testing public
health theories. (Anthropology similarly used the colonies, with its
'extremes' of behaviour.) Kenya was a colonial laboratory for testing deficiency diseases; Margaret Mellanby used it for diet and tooth decay. The
anthropologist, Audrey Richards, from her research on the Bemba
(Zambia) claimed that 'colonial malnutrition' was a modern epidemic. (It
must be also noted that African famines predate European colonisation.)
Much governmental public health was focused, protecting primarily the
health of whites and the African workers in mines and the plantations;
rural health of women and children were neglected. Whites were often
repatriated to colder climates (England) to recover, especially from mental
illness. It is interesting to note that the NHS until recently had a similar
policy of repatriation for Blacks suffering from mental illness. Jamaicans
were sent to Belleview Mental Hospital, for example.

Summarising, McKeown (1976, 1979) argued that the main improvement
in health, as evaluated by a declining mortality from infectious diseases,

was from public health interventions – improved nutrition, water safety and changes in personal behaviour. Future health profiles, although England was a 'modern society' in the 1970s, would still be dependent on an individual's behaviour – diet, smoking and exercise. The mortality rates started falling from the nineteenth century, before key vaccination programmes for TB, measles, polio and successful antibiotics for pneumonia and influenza. McKeown, however, primarily fails to explain how, although there is increased longevity for males and females there remains a five year gap, the women living longer (1998, male 74.9 and female 79.8 years). This is a demographic feature of major industrial societies. Also, focusing on mortality overrides other powerful public health ratings – as with chronicity: despite increased longevity, the years free from limiting, long-term illness has changed only slightly. In addition, McKeown gives little recognition to some doctors' participation in the public health changes. McKeown could not be expected to have commented upon the recent rise in prenatal deaths, with miscarriages; this also included pregnancy terminations. The latter has not been considered a public health issue, except indirectly related to 'under age' and teenage pregnancy rates.

What Is New About the Public Health Movement?

That we talk of a new social movement presupposes there is clear differentiation from the old, that is, they are two separate entities. The issue is complicated: there is no general agreement on what 'is' a social movement. Saint Simon (1760–1825), the French 'positivist' and social evolutionist, first used the term as a means for bringing about a new 'scientific age'. It is usually an alliance of different people who seek some aspect of social change. A movement is not as tightly organised as a political party, with its internal discipline of membership, but often has links with parties. They can be narrowly focused, as with the Thalidomide Society, and international with the globalisation movements. Cohen (1985) distinguishes between resource mobilisation, common in North America, and identity orientated movements, common in Europe. The old and new movements have in common mixed memberships, from political figures, health professions (last century mainly doctors) and some benevolent middle classes. The new have more nurses and lay clients, some politically active. Both movements regard good health and safe environment as an extension of citizens' rights. Both regard appropriate diets/food as essential for maintaining the moral order. The nineteenth-century movement was more concerned with product adulteration and that of the twentieth century with safe levels of cholesterol, additives and fats, and so on. In 1900

Salford had the 'Poison Beer' scandal when 107 people died of arsenic poisoning. Caramel used to colour mild beer was contaminated with iron pyrites, producing arsenic oxide. The Camelford water pollution (1988), when 20 tons of aluminium sulphate was added, indicates that human errors are still possible. However, the distinction between food and medicine is often blurred. Smith (2001:171) exemplifies the latter by recounting how coffee was the most frequently analysed commodity in the Lancet's Analytical Sanitary Commission Reports on adulterations 1851–54. As a result of the development of microscopical techniques the public health discourse could now rely on universal, precise measurements. (The sale of impure coffee actually dates from 1718 legislation.) The medical, nutritional and moral claims for coffee often appeared in temperance literature. The medical claims for coffee covered indigestion relief, mental stimulation (especially for craftsmen) and 'constitutional restoration' (especially from the added milk).

Lay Beliefs and Public Health

We are all able to offer explanatory accounts of health and illness. The explanations offered are often called 'lay beliefs' and are commonly at variance with the explanations produced by the bio-scientific model of the sick role used by doctors. From an early age children begin to learn the 'causation' of illness. Mothers tell children not to go out with wet hair, or to wear a vest, lest they 'catch a cold'. Unless public health specialists are able to appreciate and make sense of lay beliefs, their health promotion models will remain limited.

The new public health launched as the Public Health Alliance (1987), was a patchwork coalition of the 'left' with a new agenda. The old Labour had been out of office for almost a decade and didn't look like immediately returning. The action brought together the Trade Unions, community action groups, local authorities, the voluntary sector and ethnic-based interest together with sympathetic health workers, for example, some radical GPs. After Labour's third election defeat in 1987 it realised that 'classical' class action to reduce inequalities had rapidly faded. The collapse of the Soviet bloc reinforced this view. The much-concealed Black Report (1980) on health inequalities had little chance of being operationalised by the Conservatives. The new public health shifted health responsibility from the individual to the social. The WHO Alma Ata declaration (1978), 'Health for All by 2000', was adopted by the new public health, The Lisbon Healthy City initiatives was also another plank. The new public health was more global in policy than its old counterpart. The new public health practitioners are part of the service class (which did not exist last century). They work within the ideological state apparatus. They are concerned with the circulation of health resources as well as being consumers of it in their own right. Their targets are state given, for example, the *NHS Plan and Saving Lives: Our Healthier Nation* (DoH, 2000). In all, Labour has set out over six hundred health targets (for example, to reduce the death rate from cancer in people under 75 by at least 20 per cent by 2011). This followed the target style of the Conservatives in their Health of the Nation (DoH, 1992), introduced with little consultation from the medical profession. The primordial contract of the individual emerging from the multifarious health targets is that of the one-dimensional individual – holism has been lost with the body and self fragmented into health target areas.

Williams (1983) unravelled the lay logic of health held by early Aberdonians (over sixty years) in middle and working class estates. Both believed that 'strength' was an important constituent, a property that could be stored for future use, thereby minimising the effects of impending illness. If it was dissipated, then the capacity for quick recovery would be lost. The Protestant ethic ideologically, too, emphasises 'conservation'. 'Fitness' is the second constituent of health. The young are super-fit – fit for anything. The elderly consider themselves fit for specific activities, for example, shopping, gardening or being able to climb stairs. A third constituent of health is absence of disease. Pain was an indicator of this. Health specialists telling the aged to be highly mobile runs counter to their belief of storing good health for the winter with its potential illness crises. Other strategies to get the elderly to exercise have to be used like entertainment – social dancing, and so on.

The bio-medical model regards lay beliefs as erroneous, trivial, subjective (as opposed to 'universal' scientific knowledge). Lay beliefs are held by the majority; invoked to answer the 'why me' question which doctors avoid. Paradoxically, when the medical model cannot produce scientific explanations it also smuggles into the consultation its own lay beliefs – for example, the mysterious 'virus x' to explain ME as a 'post viral infection'. Pilgrim and Rogers (1998: 67) argue that there are epistemological grounds for doctors 'following' some lay beliefs (they were concerned primarily with psychiatry). Lay accounts are an important resource for understanding the patient's social context, producing valuable, family knowledge to aid diagnosis, and so on, 'thus lay knowledge and expert knowledge are mutually dependent and should not be studied in isolation from one another'. On the whole lay beliefs form part of an external health belief model – the causation of illness is 'out there'; the bio-scientific model is primarily an internal model – causation within the body. However, when the internal model exhausts its explanations it does not hesitate to scour the 'external environment' for an illness linkage, like stress as a cancer causation. Many ancient health beliefs, for example, Chinese or Ayervedic medicine, are primarily external health belief models.

The Future for Public Health

The future for public health is both challenging and promising in terms of the scope for development of the public health movement and the many possible difficulties it faces. The Secretary of State for Public Health, in a lecture at the London School of Economics, 8 March 2000 commented: 'The time has come to take public health out of the ghetto' (Public Health, Select Committee, 2001:14). The minister argued further that its problems were forcing it to equate with the medical model. Public health as a movement faces enormous challenges and criticisms. One of its central planks is the notion of 'empowerment', which may be seen as a piece of rhetoric which uses the idea of power sharing by providing health recipients with choices but which in practice reinforces an existing paternalistic relationship.

There are numerous changes taking place in public health which are yet to develop into effective policy initiatives (Select Committee 2001:21), such as the development of the Health Development Agency (HDA), Health Action Zones (HAZ), Health Improvement Programmes (HIP), Health Living Centres (HLC), Public Health Observatories (PHO), Health Impact Assessment (HIA) and the National Institute of Clinical Excellence (NICE). Reflecting on these numerous initiatives, it may be argued that New Labour could be accused of 'initiative overload'. The Reporting of the Chief Medical Officer (2001) and Select Committee called for public health to cohere the fragmented NHS structure. There are parallels here with the Barclay Report (1982) with its idealistic design for social work to orchestrate community interests and organisations into a seamless service. The challenge for public health is to establish 'strong partnerships' at all levels for a broad-based approach to public health (p. 120). A new style of 'strong leadership' will be required with the need to build the evidence-based practice. Health policy should benefit the less well off on a sliding scale rather than targeting the most deprived (p. 127). Local leadership should also be involved. The Chief Medical Officer's Report goes over much the same territory and suggests 'strengthening the public health skills' ... 'working alongside clinicians' ... 'to meet needs' (p. 37) ... 'strengthen the multidisciplinary' nature of the public health and PCG/T. There should also be provision for GPs to gain training in public health and have correspondingly a relevant career structure. There should also be a three-year rolling public health development plan for education, training and organisational development covering different sections of the public health workforce

(p. 29). The Select Committee ends by stating that the Government must learn the lessons of previous policy, 'particularly with regard to political leadership and commitment making health improvements a central priority' (p. 136). With its public health proposals, as a prescriptive exercise, it is limited. It fails to give details of much of the operationalisation thrust needed. It assumes 'strong leadership' (undefined); and 'joint partnerships' (undefined) are talisman. The tacit rules of the organisational settings are totally neglected. Giving public health a networking function to cohere disparate health organisations may appear pictographically neat in future health documents, but that does mean a new 'health synthesis' has been achieved. To increase the professional status of public health with new higher degrees and the creation of the new Health Development Agency and Public Health Observatories may actually increase the inter-professional rivalries already existing in health delivery. The Select Committee's suggestion that the NHS Executive Regional Offices can take a greater strategic role in public health (p. 136) may be the catalyst for its networking. Much depends on the Government's serious intent of raising the profile economically and clinically of primary health care at the expense of the entrenched hospital base.

Conclusion

In conclusion, it may be seen that public health historically has come a long way in the last decade and as health care has become more complex so too has the design and delivery of health services. The chapter set out to open up public health debates for the reader to see how far and how much the movement has progressed. In the following chapters the reader is exposed to the many social and individual issues influencing public health (Chapter 2) and asked to consider the relationship between the underlying causation of illness such as social class differences (Chapter 3) and poverty in order to develop a fuller appreciation of those factors contributing towards public health. Taking into account the multicultural nature of modern society Costello *et al.* in Chapter 4 examine and debate the health needs of diverse ethnic groups and the needs of those seen to be vulnerable in our society (Chapter 5). Chapter 6 considers the way in which media portrayals of health can provide and help to construct a distorted image of health as we struggle to develop a clear picture of what health is. Maria Horne, in Chapter 7, takes us through the process of assessing health needs by focusing on community health issues and the public health assessment strategies used to develop ways of meeting need for large populations. In Chapter 8 Costello's examination of the political implications of public health describes and analyses the work of the Government's Social Exclusion Units, introducing the reader to the ways in which social change is taking place from a political perspective. In the final chapter, Haggart considers the role of public health nursing and assesses the future of public health from the viewpoint of practitioners who take responsibility for the health of individuals and families.

References

Ashton, J. and Seymour, H. (1988) *The New Public Health*. Buckingham: Open University Press.

Barclay, R. (The Barclay Report) (1982) *Social Workers: Their Role and Tasks*. London: National Institute for Social Work.

Black Report (1980) *Inequalities of Health, Report of a Research Working Group*, Chairman Sir Douglas Black. London: DHSS (published in 1982 by Pelican Press).

Brockington, F. (1960) *The Health of Community Principles: Public Health for Practitioners and Students* (2nd edn). London: JA Churchill.

Burls, A. (2000) Public participation in public health decisions. In Bradley, P. and Burls, A. (eds) *Ethics in Public and Community Health*. London: Routledge.

Cohen, J.L. (1985) Strategy or identity: new medical paradigms and contemporary social movements. *Social Research*, 52, 663–716.

DoH (Department of Health) (1992) *The Health of the Nation*. London: HMSO.

DoH (Department of Health) (2000) *The NHS Plan. A Plan for Investment A Plan for Reform*. London, CM 4818.1.

DoH (Department of Health) (2001) The report of the CMO's *Project to Strengthen the Public Health Function*. London: DoH.

Dossey, B. (2000) *Florence Nightingale: Mystic, Visionary, Healer*. New York: Springhouse.

Engels, F. (1982) *Conditions of the Working Classes in England in 1844*. London: Allen and Unwin.

Farr, M. (1836) *Philosophy of Health*, London: Constable.

Griffiths, S. and Hunter, D.J. (1999) *Perspectives in Public Health*. Oxford: Radcliffe Medical Press.

Hamlin, C. (2000) Public health and social justice. In *The age of Chadwick: Britain 1800–1854*. Cambridge, UK: Cambridge University Press.

Harrison, M. (1994) *The Public Health in British India 1859–1914*. Cambridge: Cambridge University Press.

Hillery, G.A. (1996) Definitions of community: Areas of agreement. *Rural Sociology*, 21, 111–23.

Health Committee (2001) Second Report, Public Health Vol 1 (March 19), Report and Proceedings of the Committee. London: HMSO.

Illich, I. (1976) *Medical Nemesis – The Expropriation of Health*. London: Marion Boyars.

Lalonde, E. (1974) *New Perspective on the Health of Canadians*. Ottowa: Ministry Supply and Services.

Le Fanu , J. (1999) *Rise and Fall of Modern Medicine*. London: Little Brown Co.

McKeown, T. (1976) *The Modern Rise of Population*. London: Edward Arnold.

McKeown, T. (1979) *The Role of Medicine*. Oxford: Basil Blackwell.

Nightingale, F. (1860) *Notes on Nursing: What it is and What it is Not*. London: Harrison.

Pilgrim, D. and Rogers, A. (1998) The wisdom of lay knowledge: A reply to Loughlin and Prichard. *Health Care Analysis*, 6, 65–71.

Porter, R. (1997) *The Greatest Benefit to Mankind: A Medical History of Humanity from Antiquity to the Present*. London: HarperCollins.

Richman, J. (1987) *Medicine and health*. London: Longman.

Rosen, G. (1993) *A History of Public Health*. Baltimore: John Hopkins University Press.

Small, H. (1998) *Florence Nightingale Avenging Angel*. London: Constable.

Smith, S.D. (2001) Coffee, microscopy, and the Lancet's Analytical Sanitary Commission. *Social History of Medicine*, 14, 171–97.

Sontag, S. (1979) *Illness as a Metaphor*. London: Allen Lane.
Tonnies, F. (1957) *Community and Society*. New York: Harper Row.
Ward, D. (1972) In Freeman, H.E., Levine, S. and Reeder, L.G. (eds) *The Handbook of Sociology*.
    Prentice Hall: New Jersey.
WHO (1952) Inaugural meeting of World Health Organisation. Geneva: WHO.
Williams, R. (1983) The concepts of health: An analysis of lay logic. *Sociology*, 17, 185–205.

2

Social and Individual Factors Influencing Public Health

RON IPHOFEN

On the whole, we are meant to look after ourselves; it is certain each has to eat for himself, digest for himself, and in general care for his own dear life, and see to his own preservation; nature's intentions, in most things uncertain, in this are decisive. (Arthur Hugh Clough, 1819–1861)

The key points discussed in this chapter include:

- the influence of socio-economic status on the health of the general public
- how the factors which influence health differ according to a range of circumstances
- how health promotion information can be used to improve the health and life chances for all.

Introduction

Most health professionals know the comprehensive sociological research evidence linking poor health to social background factors. Hierarchies of age, gender, housing, ethnicity, education and social class are linked to health and illness and the evidence of this relationship has been regularly confirmed in a succession of studies (see Brocklehurst and Costello, Chapter 3 and Marmot and Wilkinson, 1999). Those 'low down' on the social class hierarchy, with little formal education and from economically deprived groups have worse housing, are less well fed, less fit and more likely to engage in commonplace 'risky' health behaviours. As a consequence these are the people most found in need of health service support and are most likely to become ill and die sooner. But health professionals

are also well aware that every one of their clients is unique and too broad
a generalisation about their situation does a disservice to their special
qualities and individual problems.

The purpose of this chapter is to explore the background to these well-
established observations in order to inform health professionals in their
attempts to do something about the health of the general public. In practical terms the questions are: how do those factors, which influence us all,
differ in the way in which they combine to influence each of us?, and how
can that information be used to improve the health and life chances for all?

In this respect, the chapter links to the recurrent themes of this book –
how professionals can empower the public to seek and maintain better
health as well as enhancing their control over these apparently implacable
relationships between the health of individuals and their place in the
social structure.

The Influence of Social Structure

Research and writing in this field is extensive. Albrecht *et al.* (2000) sum-
marise a range of social influences on public health. It is indisputable that
variations in health status are linked to socio-economic differences
between individuals, communities and societies, and that such inequalities persist in spite of global economic and social development (Robert
and House, 2000). Although such correlations have been observed for
some time, a full understanding of the mechanisms connecting material
and cultural conditions and the health behaviours of individuals, communities and societies has still to be achieved.

All the evidence available from a range of studies documents that
higher rates of morbidity and mortality and of functional and mental disabilities coincide with lower levels of education, income, occupation,
material resources and home ownership (Williams, 1990; Acheson, 1998).
This relationship is quite complex since there are difficulties associated
with the measurement of both socio-economic position and of health
status (Marmot *et al.*, 1997). This presents a fundamental problem for
social epidemiology. Health and illness are not dichotomous, they vary in
their distribution across a population and within individuals. Groups and
individuals are not *either* healthy *or* diseased, they are 'more or less'
healthy, and that relative health varies according to a range of social background characteristics (Iphofen and Poland, 1998:248–51). Causality is not,
of course, determined by mere correlation, and the pattern of relationship
between health outcomes and background social factors is even more
complicated within the different levels of the social status hierarchy
(Robert and House, 2000:116–20).

This complication is well demonstrated when using, say, 'level of education attained' as an indicator of social status. There is a strong correlation between education and good health and an improved sense of well-being in the individual. Part of the explanation for this may be that since university graduates, for example; take a more proactive rather than reactive approach to life, they are better able to handle crisis and change. They are more likely to adopt preventive approaches to illness and have increased self-confidence and motivation. Perhaps as a consequence they are less likely to have to face general mental health problems. However, on the down side, more highly educated people are more vulnerable to chronic fatigue syndrome and some eating disorders. Women graduates also have an increased likelihood of divorce and the children of graduates are more likely to have allergies and atopic disabilities (Bynner and Egerton, 2001).

It is only when each of the social indicators is examined in detail that we can see the complex links between health outcomes. Thus, while it is *generally* the case that education improves health status it is not so in *all* aspects of the health experience of individuals.

Even at the societal level, research suggests that, for developed countries, the bigger the gap in income between rich and poor, the poorer the health of the population (Wilkinson, 1996). Also, within such countries regional variations in income inequality correspond to variations in health status (Lynch and Kaplan, 1997). This suggests that it is not absolute differences in income or wealth that directly influence health status – such as through access to material resources – but the relative *perceptions* of income and wealth variations within the population.

Methodological Problems

Evidence of the correlations between health and social background discussed above is invariably gained from populations, not from people. By that is meant that the evidence is gained from the recorded behaviour of groups, not from the actions of the separate individuals who make up those groups. In part this explains why the generic evidence links smoking to cancer and other diseases while many people know someone who has smoked throughout their lives and suffered no apparent consequences and dies of 'natural' causes at a ripe old age. The generic evidence does not help to explain why some individuals manage to 'escape' the influence of background social factors.

The problem is that the outcome measures (of health status) and the social indicators (of social class, home ownership, age, education and so on) are collected and reported as percentages and averaged across groups, communities or societies. Such averages are therefore measures that convey information about a group, not about the individuals who make up the group. Thus, for measurement reasons, the public health 'evidence' that is acquired from populations may be divorced from the actual experiences of health and illness in the individuals who make up the phenomenon.

Failure to appreciate this methodological problem accounts for why the interests, concerns and data of public health and those of health promotion (and even health education) might have been at odds with each other. Most health professionals in practice do their work with individuals, not with groups. Even when they work with groups they target the problems of the individuals within them. For this reason the explanatory focus should rest upon the detailed examination of the linkages between individual action and social location. What permits or enables people to take action about their health?

Power and Political Resources

People only take action if they have the desire and the power to do so. Power is the ability to achieve goals even if others obstruct or attempt to prevent one from doing so. Being powerful depends upon having access to political resources – the means of persuading others to do what one would like them to do. Such resources include material resources (such as wealth, income and property), knowledge, information, physical force and so on (see Iphofen and Poland, 1998:18–30). In fact, these very resources are some of the things being measured as the social indicators that link to poor health outcome. That is like saying that people have poor health because they lack access to the things that would allow them to seek good health – a simple truism.

But what this means for public health is that political resources would need to be applied to ensure that individuals, communities and societies are able to gain access to the means for achieving healthy living. This would include information about health and access to services dedicated to caring for people when they are ill. Individuals would be best able to control their own health if they held such power. The political backcloth to individual decisions lies in the messages people receive from government, balanced against the messages they receive from family, community and society in general. Mostly for economic and political reasons governments of all persuasions in recent years have focused on the idea of the individual, family and community taking responsibility for health. Resources for health will always be limited, but all governments are sensitive to the charge that they may not be doing enough about health. As a consequence they tend to advocate individuals doing more to help themselves.

Margaret Thatcher's Government, for example; helped to establish a modern creed of individuality that has been seen as encouraging self-interested behaviour. As Prime Minister, Tony Blair has focused on the need for families to recognise their own care obligations – something entirely consistent with Thatcherite politics. Thatcher, however, famously denied the existence of society, while Blair has advocated communitarianism (Etzioni, 1993), a form of action which ties group responsibility to a geographical locality. This is not inconsistent with the need for individuals to take action on their own behalf since Amitai Etzioni (and Blair) both acknowledge the importance of individual actions in the achievement of community. As a consequence of such philosophies all the Department of Health (DoH) policy documents produced in the last two decades of the twentieth century have laid stress on the need for increased individual responsibility for health improvement. The role of the State has tended to be one of ensuring adequate health service provision for illness – not necessarily for health. The individual is then treated as a 'service consumer' whose measured 'satisfaction' becomes a key criterion of service success.

What such a policy does is to ignore background social inequalities in opportunity, assume everyone accesses the health service from the same starting-point, and measures efficiency in terms of the effectiveness of dealing with illness and not with the health gains of individuals. Necessarily, the vocabulary of central government attempted to disguise this neglect. The Conservative Government refused to use the phrase 'health inequality' and DoH documents at the time used the phrase 'health variations'. Other policies spoke of 'health improvement' and 'health gain', both of which were measured in terms of illness reduction – less cancer, less heart disease and so on. During this period no government fundamentally addressed the resources needed by individuals to improve their own health.

So, if individuals are to be able to do more for themselves there needs to be a social and political framework which encourages and facilitates access to health-related resources. Unfortunately it continues to be the case that, at the societal level, fundamental socially structured differences in access to resources seem to persist.

The Influence of Culture

Much of the evidence identifies cultural influences as particularly dominant in health choices and chances. Thus, while social class may be measured by occupational status, the more direct influence on human action is the pressure upon thoughts and action about health behaviours that comes from the direct influences of workplace and home life (Williams, 1983; Gray, 2001: 235–56). In this way 'peer pressure' becomes a strong determinant of health behaviours.

The influence of culture is brought home when one thinks about how different sorts of people seek health in different ways. Thus there are strong variations between the type of people who seek to keep fit by playing football and those who choose to practice yoga, or between those who play rugby and those who engage in tai chi. Similarly, while most of us might conventionally visit a GP, fewer will seek help from an acupuncturist and fewer still decide to have colonic irrigation.

We can illustrate the power of cultural influences where they are perhaps strongest: in food tastes and dietary choices. Food is not merely used to provide us with nutrition and enable our physical survival; its production, distribution and consumption is culturally grounded. Consuming food in particular is more than a nutritional event; it may be social, cultural, economic, psychological and even political. Food consumption marks out daily routines, it is essential to celebration, may be part of religious ceremony, routine social interactions and exceptional occasions. The use and distribution of food replicates and perpetuates family dynamics which are often rooted in strong local cultures (Delphy, 1979; Kerr and Charles, 1986; Bell and Valentine, 1997).

We use food to communicate. It can take on a symbolic significance (Atkinson, 1979). Sometimes it is given by others as a reward or insisted upon by others (in some cultures it may be seen as impolite to refuse the gift of food). At other times we self-reward after effort. We might treat ourselves with cake or champagne, or extra helpings. Even the packaging and presentation of food is designed to entice the purchaser – convenience, nutrition, taste, or luxury are communicated in the package and enhanced by added ingredients. Thus attraction to food may be determined by our own values, needs and priorities – all factors recognised by those making and selling food (see, for example; Mennel, 1985; Mennel *et al.*, 1992).

Similarly a 'diet' is not just about weight reduction. Our diet is the combination of foodstuffs that are routinely eaten by a specified group or individual. A diet is a way of eating which forms a significant part of one's life-style. For example; since the 1930s there has been an active 'natural hygiene' movement – to find the means for facilitating the natural, innate process of survival. Every way we interact with our environment influences whether we facilitate or thwart our body's attempts to secure its well-being. There is little that is 'natural' about that interaction with our environment in the sense that it is automatic and unimpeded. It is mediated by how we think and the people we relate to.

Mediating Factors

What needs to be explored more fully are the mediating factors linking measured variations in health and socio-economic status. As suggested above, these seem to be connected to material resource deprivation, inadequate physical living conditions, psychosocial risk factors and cultural variations in health-related behaviours, knowledge and attitudes. But this is clearly not the whole story.

There is some suggestion, for example; that *sensed relative deprivation* within social hierarchies has more of an effect on health outcomes (Sapolsky, 1994; Marmot *et al.*, 1997). More needs to be done to clarify how perceptions of, say, unfair treatment or disadvantage directly affect human cognition, emotion and behaviour. It is ironic that some of those most disadvantaged in society, in terms of physical or learning disability, have low levels of resentment or sensed injustice about their restricted opportunities. Some argue that social cohesion or 'trust' is a key explanatory variable explaining the phenomenon (Robert and House, 2000:126). Kawachi and Kennedy (1997) even offer evidence of measured correlations between population mortality, lack of trust in people and low tolerance of income inequality.

What mediates between a central governmental (or even global) policy decision to target particular health goals is the fact that it is the individuals who possess the thoughts and attitudes and perform the behaviour that make the attainment of such goals possible. If individuals choose not to act in response to those cherished goals, they will not be achieved.

Individual Action

All of the above does suggest the need for a more careful examination of individual responses to social influences. In other words, subjective perceptions of differences in social status may be more significant than objective measures of structural location.

Individual responsibility has been eroded over many centuries within the Western Christian tradition. Large institutions have steadily assumed more power and control over the lives of individuals. These institutions include the social control agencies of medicine, religion and the State (Illich, 1977; Foucault, 1980). The nature of such institutional power is better understood when contrasted with alternative cultural traditions. In Muslim and in Buddhist philosophy, for example; it can only be individuals who make decisions, take actions and, necessarily, bear the consequences of those actions. The notion of a 'welfare state' has little place in such traditions.

The taking of responsibility by an individual or group depends upon a range of interacting factors. In practice, it may be difficult to understand their separate influences upon an individual's or group's ability and willingness to take responsibility for their health. To examine these influences in detail it is necessary first to separate them out and then to examine their interdependence.

In health terms, the most vital factors are *needs*. These are things that cannot be done without. They represent the essential means for survival or maintenance of the body – the nutrients and energy sources we require from food and the environment. Professionals should know about such things, but individuals may not be best placed to recognise their own needs, since they frequently confuse them with 'wants'. Wants are things we could do without but would like to have to make life more pleasant, interesting or whatever. We might want our regular cup of cappuccino, or bar of chocolate, but we don't need them to live.

Ability is a major factor in individual empowerment – we cannot take responsibility if we cannot act. It is in this element that political resources are vital. We need skills, competencies and resources that enable us to take action to remedy, improve and sustain health. But we also have to *value* whatever it is we are taking responsibility for. If we are to be responsible for learning, then learning has to be important to us. If we are to be responsible for our health (or the health of someone else) then health has to be valued. We may do this because human life *per se* is valued, or that 'looking good' and being fit is important to us. We may even believe that it is wrong not to care for our own body, or wrong to allow others not to care for theirs, and so on. In this way health even becomes a moral issue (see Brandt and Rozin, 1997).

Of course, we also have to *believe* or make the assumption that our actions can make a difference to health or that the *knowledge* we are applying is accurate. Knowledge is another vital factor. We have to know how to act, why we are acting in a particular way and, therefore, we need access to the information which allows us that knowledge. Finally, we need the will to act – we need *motivation*. To be motivated to seek and maintain health, we must want to *take responsibility* for it.

To assess the propensity for individuals or groups to take action with regard to their health, then, one could apply the following check-list:

- needs
- wants
- ability
- values

- beliefs
- knowledge
- motives.

One would then need to examine the way in which these factors are mutually interdependent. Thus, understanding our needs is evidently dependent upon our knowledge of our body – how it works, what happens when things go wrong and how these things might be rectified. In the same way, we need knowledge of our society, our community and family and how these influence our wants, values, motives, and so on. Wants depend upon feelings, emotions, attitudes and preferences and so are linked to values and assumptions.

Abilities are linked to knowledge – we are not able to act if we do not know how to act or why we should act in particular ways. Motivation is also linked to resources (such as time and ability) as well as to values and assumptions – such as a belief in the possibility of a successful outcome. In other words, it helps to believe that our efforts will, in fact, make a difference to our health.

Costs and Benefits to Individuals and to Groups

One way to examine the socio-cultural and structural influences upon the health of individuals and groups is to use the factors check-listed above and examine the kinds of rational cost/benefit analyses that people routinely engage in when they take action – or neglect to – about their health. In other words, it is necessary to explore what facilitates and what inhibits the taking of personal responsibility for health and the taking of health risks.

Food and diet once again provide an excellent focus for personal cost/benefit analyses since they are so taken for granted as part of our way of life that sometimes we forget to ask the key health-related questions about them. We should be asking why we eat what we eat, why certain foods are produced and not others, how foods are produced and what ingredients are added to food and for what purpose (Sokolov, 1991). Concern over ingredients is a balance of needs and wants against values and resources. How much time do you have to find things out and how much does it matter? Does food labelling help or hinder? Is it an inconvenience of daily life to have to wade through the ingredients listed on a food package, or is it essential for our ability to protect and improve our own health?

It is only in recent years that, as a consequence of a series of food crises such as salmonella in eggs, BSE and GM foods that public awareness and concern has grown to such an extent that the production and marketing of food has had to be modified to account for changes in public consumption. Thus the range of vegan, vegetarian and organic foods has grown immensely in the last few years as the major suppliers have responded to the economic pressures of market demands. The Government established the Food Standards Agency in response to public concern and even a food labelling initiative in 2001.

A more telling example is provided in attitudes to the drinking of water. The British public appear to have a taste for fluids that are canned, sweetened, carbonated, commercially packaged, advertised and/or ultimately dehydrating, such as tea, coffee, soft drinks and alcohol. Public knowledge of the importance of pure water and how it should be consumed daily by individuals for their better health is abysmal. The body of a person weighing 10 stone (65 kilos) contains about 40 litres of water. On a cool day that person should take in at least eight big glasses of water to meet their body's requirements. In fact, the neglect of our body's need for re-hydration is so great that we often even fail to recognise 'thirst' any more and confuse it with hunger (Batmanghelidj, 2000). Water from the tap is taken for granted and its 'ingredients' rarely questioned, even those who know of the need to consume adequate amounts of water frequently neglect to do so – even though the environments in which we live and work are increasingly dehydrating. Car travel, central heating, TV screens and VDUs are all liable to increase our need for water and yet it is still something that is rarely provided as a routine part of our living and working environment. Restaurants in the USA automatically place a jug of water and glasses on the table as you take your seat, it has to be requested in British restaurants. How many workplaces routinely offer easy access to filtered drinking water?

To understand why people do not alter their behaviour with something as simple as drinking water, it is necessary to examine the cost/benefit analyses we sometimes knowingly, but more often subconsciously, conduct. It is much the same process as the 'balance of risks'. Some risks are known and disclosed; others less known or deliberately concealed. Responsibility (collective or individual) must shift according to the available personal evidence. Once the knowledge is gained, how easy is it to maintain the behaviour? What are the consequences on other aspects of our lives, such as the increased frequency of urination, or the easy availability of acceptable drinking water at home, at recreational sites or at work? Do some of these things simply take too much effort?

So there are contrasting inhibiting factors which counteract the individual or combined effects of the background influences of culture or social structure. There are mechanisms which stop or discourage people from both gaining knowledge or accessing information, or even having the desire to gain such knowledge. These mechanisms include the hypnotic effects of advertising and the dominance of particular cultural views leading to an acceptance of the status quo. To understand how this happens we must ask further analytical questions such as:

• Who invests in maintaining such 'acceptances'?

• Who monopolises constructions of images related to health behaviour?

• Who invests in stopping people wanting to gain knowledge?

Clearly, the manufacturers, distributors and advertisers of products that influence our health have a vested interest in public ignorance. Only in that way can they encourage the public to buy products that may be of no health benefit and may even do harm. The balance of dominant cultural messages in the mass media in favour of 'less healthy' options is difficult for professionals to intervene in without major economic resources (see King, Chapter 6). Public health is not directly profitable to commercial interests, so ways have to be found to utilise mass media which might not be so costly in terms of resources (Atkin and Wallack, 1990).

Examining the disincentives to taking responsibility for health can be quite surprising. 'Inconvenience' is clearly a sufficient disincentive for action for some people – it is a 'cost'. For others there may be clear advantages to 'not being healthy'. For example; it might be difficult for the young and healthy to conceive of any positive aspects of being old or being infirm, and yet even small things might be conceived of as 'trade-off' benefits, such as having a disabled car parking sticker and being able to park anywhere in town. Most health professionals will be aware of the secondary gains from being ill – that others will, up to a point, have more sympathy and provide care and attention. Most people will have heard comments like 'I know that smoking makes me ill/is bad for me/is killing me, but it certainly helps me relax/is the only pleasure I have ...' and so on (see Graham, 1993).

By analysing an individual or group's characteristics (such as needs and wants) and then relating them to their personal cost/benefit analyses, we might gain insight into health-related attitudes and behaviour. But there is a danger in connecting this directly to blame and accountability. How can we blame someone who is unhealthy through their own lack of knowledge, whose beliefs and values are at variance with ours and who lacks the ability to remedy this deficiency? One doesn't have to look far for examples of how difficult these issues are to reconcile. For example; who is responsible for any damage if a person takes a toxic drug knowing that there is a risk with it? What if they do not know there is a risk, but someone else does? What is the likelihood of the 'someone else' getting the necessary information to them? What if the person did not take all reasonable steps to find out that risk, and the 'knowing' other deliberately took steps to conceal the known risk?

This is exactly what happened in the case of cigarette smoking. It is now well known that the tobacco companies withheld information about the dangers of smoking. But even after the evidence was overwhelming, people have continued to smoke. At first advertising and popular culture 'normalised' the behaviour and now, since mass advertising has been stopped, smoking has taken on some of the characteristics of the 'rebellious youth' subculture – encouraging a shared defensiveness among young smokers.

The problem then becomes whether individuals are concerned about maintaining their health to such an extent that reducing health risks reduces the quality of their life. To use another example: in some respects the world has always been a 'dangerous' place but parents today are more aware of the dangers to their children and discourage them from a range of 'risky' activities. These include walking to school on their own, playing in certain places, being in traffic, and so on – all activities that were once an integral part of learning about life. Even technology designed to improve our life-style can influence our health. Modern tennis racquets, for example; enable the ball to be hit harder and are so light that we are more liable to make incorrect strikes of the ball that can damage elbows and wrist. The boxing glove is a classic example of a technological improvement with enhanced risk. Bare-knuckle fights were always much shorter and with less damage done since the fighters' knuckles would get so cut and bruised that they couldn't continue. The boxing glove enables the fight to go on so long that the likelihood of brain damage from successive blows to the head is increased (see Tenner, 1996).

Public Health Policy

To think in terms of managing the balance between individual and collective responsibility might help us to understand some of the problems we face in meeting the demands of a modern health care system.

The policy questions, put simply, are: How much should individuals do – or could be expected to do to maintain their health? How much should/must the State do either at the institutional level or via its agents?

Public health at the societal level can provide the much-needed material resource infrastructure. Public health policy has to find ways to redress the persistent observed inequalities in health status while lacking the ability – perhaps because of a failure of political will – to alter the fundamental social differentiation upon which they are based. Public health agents rarely possess the power, let alone the right, to interfere in the public's decision to seek or not to seek health, to take or not to take health risks. Moreover, as political institutions stand, public health *per se* has lacked the political leverage that, say, the DoH or the NHS possesses overall and, certainly in the eyes of the Treasury, commands much less attention.

It has long been the case historically that governments become interested in public health only when there is sufficient economic justification for doing so and when it becomes politically expedient to be seen to intervene. With the incoming 1997 Labour Government there was awareness that there could be some distinct political capital to be gained from public health improvement. One survey found that of the 100 constituencies with the worst health, 97 were Labour, and of the 100 constituencies with the best health, 81 were Conservative – thus confirming the link between wealth and health (assuming the wealthy are still more likely to be Tory supporters) (Laurance, 2001:35). By reducing the health gap between rich and poor, Labour could have a vote winner. The succession of policies aimed at reducing social inequality generally and specifically in the health field can be justified as a consequence of this awareness: the Social Exclusion Unit (see Costello, Chapter 8), the New Deal, and Welfare to Work were designed to address social inequality. Health Action Zones and 'healthy living centres' aimed to remove inter-agency barriers between health and social care.

It is clear that public health policy can only accomplish health improvement goals if it addresses change at all levels, from the individual to the global. Policies aimed at reducing social inequality could be seen to have some health improvement consequences for the most disadvantaged sectors of the population (Mitchell *et al.*, 2001). Despite its range of policies to redress health inequality (the establishment of the Health Development Agency and regional public health observatories) the current Labour Government has no plans to redistribute income from the rich to the poor even though the gap is widening. Some estimates suggest that returning income differentials to what they were in 1983 could save 10,000 people between the ages of 16 and 64 from premature death and 1,400 children under 15 from avoidable mortality (Laurance, 2001:37). Politically and economically addressing these fundamental resource and life-style issues remains a less viable policy than encouraging enhanced individual responsibility.

At the communal level an approach that does bear some merit appears to be based on improvements in social capital. It is possible that interventions targeting social engagement and social networks (Berkman *et al.*, 2000) could help reduce the chronic anxiety, sensed insecurity, social isolation and perceived lack of control that contribute to undermining mental and physical health (Brunner and Marmot, 1999). In any case, it appears that the underlying mediating factors and individuals' own cost/benefit analyses and estimates of risk are more persistent influences than the indirect consequences of socio-economic position (see, for example; House *et al.*, 1990; Williams, 1990; Link and Phelan, 1995).

Thus it is generally accepted that improved access to medical care will not alone rectify the fundamental imbalance in health outcomes (Robert and House, 2000:121). In fact, curiously, there is evidence to suggest that reduced access to medical care can improve a population's health chances. When doctors went on strike for a month in Israel in 1973 admissions to hospital went down by 85 per cent and the death rate dropped by 50 per cent. When doctors went on strike in Los Angeles County in the USA in 1976 the death rate dropped by 20 per cent and returned to previous levels when the strike was over (McDermott and O'Connor, 1996:6). More recently there has been heightened public awareness of nosocomial infections acquired by patients during their hospital stay. Such infections cause prolonged illness and even death for the more vulnerable patients (Marinella *et al.*, 1997). Thus the grounds for arguing for improved health services might be questionable if it only means more of the same.

If medical treatment is so tangential to general health, then a more effective policy to address responsibility, life-style and resource problems should be implemented by shifting the balance of power in institutional health care from the NHS to other agencies. At the governmental level this could imply government departments and local authorities taking more account of how their actions can improve health chances. Similarly the education system and employers could take a bigger role in health improvement, as could the voluntary sector and leisure industry. State resources might then be more effectively redistributed to allow such agencies to work directly with individuals and groups at a local level in order to improve their health care (Laurance, 2001:38).

The state of current sociological research in not fully exploring the social influences on health behaviours and outcomes has implications for public health policy. More work needs to be done on the linkages between individual actions on health and the availability of resources within communities. The conditions of the built physical environment, its productive consequences and transportation and distribution facilities all condition access to health-related services and resources. It is evident that changing this resource base alone will not improve the health of individuals unless their beliefs, values and knowledge are also altered.

The Mediating Role of the Health Professional

As outlined earlier, health professionals stand at the coal-face of this relationship and mediate between the background social and cultural factors and the target individuals they are caring for who take (more or less) rational decisions about their health attitudes and behaviour. While professionals can be expected to have more knowledge about health risks and maintenance factors, they may have no more power to change fundamental social and communal structures than the individuals themselves.

So the question remains – what can individual health professionals do to enhance the responsible health behaviour of their clients? In essence it is connected to what defines them as 'professionals' in the first place: they have to have more knowledge and more power than their clients and to use such assets in the interests of their clients.

One pertinent area of development in recent years has become known as 'narrative-based medicine' (Greenhalgh and Hurwitz, 1999). Listening to the stories that people tell about their health and illness can illuminate the background to links between the demographics and the individual. Exploration of a narrative account can reveal more rapidly the nature of, say, eating behaviour and relative perceptions of excessive food and alcohol consumption than questionnaires or history taking can. Professionals can even use the narrative form to encourage individuals to consider alternative health behaviours; in other words, they can engage in health promotion.

The truth is, of course, that taking responsibility is hard work. Individuals need help to persist with health improvement when pressured externally by social situations. They need the time, energy and resources to allow healing to take place and/or to resist illness while they are still functioning in the world. This is true even for health professionals themselves; many nurses still smoke and many doctors drink too much alcohol. As an intelligent, well-educated and reasonably well-resourced professional, I take many active steps to maintain and improve my health – but it requires effort, time and the will to do so. I know that if an expert helped me it would facilitate the process. I cannot possibly know all the ingredients in my food choices, what their 'e' number represents or whether they are likely to have detrimental effects, but if steered to the correct literature I am better informed and thus able to act in my own best interests (Cox and Brusseau, 1997). If I decide to engage in a natural colon cleanse, I may precipitate a 'cleansing crisis' which produces illness symptoms. I would not be 'ill', since my body would be healing naturally, but I would not want it to be channelled away from an approach to health care which resonates with my cultural and personal beliefs and practices (Diamond and Diamond, 1985). I still need help, advice and guidance that is congruent with my preferred beliefs and practices – unless, of course, they have been proven to be radically erroneous. Then I need help in changing beliefs and practices about health.

To advocate taking responsibility does not necessarily mean complete self-help. Otherwise why maintain a public health service? In any case the information and help available is immense, complex and confusing. To take responsibility means to desire to maintain one's health, to avoid illness and to be more informed about symptoms and preventative measures. It means eating and drinking in a healthy manner, being more aware about one's own body, taking precautionary measures when necessary and taking fewer risks. It cannot mean being left to one's own devices. With knowledge and the possibility that help is available, people feel less fear about illness and may become more disposed to take action for their own health.

So it is also important that health professionals aiming to improve public health are neither ethnocentric nor dominated by principles of Western medicine. The general public are much more aware of complementary and alternative medicine (CAM) and seek it out increasingly (Kelner and Wellman, 1997). In a multicultural society professionals have to take responsibility for broadening their knowledge of available techniques. In this way they empower themselves and their clients. Ayurvedic principles, traditional Chinese medicine, naturopathy and herbal medicine are now generally available, along with other techniques such as acupuncture, reflexology, aromatherapy, and so on. The recent House of Lords Committee Report on Science and Technology has added legitimacy to CAM by recommending procedures for improving the evidence base and regulating the CAM professions in the same ways as other health professions.

At the societal level it is vital that health professionals make use of their own political resources to ensure that the politics of neither government nor of the health professions themselves restrict access to beneficial health support. What has been called professional 'tribalism' can impede progress in public health. While health is seen as the prerogative of any one group or agency it can be subject to trends, fashions and whatever is seen as constituting the effective 'evidence base'. Such things can change as knowledge and informed opinion change; the danger lies in narrow-mindedness and tunnel vision within a profession or discipline. If public health professionals are mindful of such tendencies they are best placed to make a difference.

Conclusion

The argument of this chapter has been that individual experiences of health and illness are frequently glossed over for the purposes of measuring the extent of the problem and thereby influencing governmental policy at the societal level. If public health is to make a difference it is through the health professionals who deal directly with individuals and groups – these are the 'means' that facilitate change – alongside the actions taken independently by those individuals. Any means to directly influence the lives and circumstances of individuals will ultimately facilitate health gain and health improvement.

It is, of course, those individuals who are the target of public health who need to take the actions that make the difference. But the seeking and maintaining of health is a relentless process. It consumes time, energy and material resources – the very resources required for its maintenance. This is why the permanently disabled or less able are constantly depleted of resources and in need of their continuous supply to maintain their health or avoid further illness. In this respect the professionals' success is only partly dependent upon individuals determined to become and remain in charge of their own health. Throughout this chapter I have been concerned to explore how and why individuals choose to take action about their health.

In a complex modern society individual responsibility is hard to achieve. In less 'developed' societies people have little choice. In all societies few individuals have all the power they need to take control even of their own lives. If individuals need to gain access to the corporate resources of public and/or private institutions they require the information and the ability to do so. The professionals' role is to make up for what individuals will necessarily lack in this regard, either as a consequence of their individual biography or of their structural and cultural location. Some people are simply better placed than others to assume individual responsibility, while those who are less 'able' must rely directly on the intervention of health professionals. If that intervention works from the societal, through the communal, to the individual level via employers, community organisations and local government, then individuals may be empowered to retreat partially or temporarily from the pressures of life while they heal and recuperate. Better still, professionals could marshal their resources and act to facilitate healthy working and living practices by intervening in the social settings where unhealthy behaviours, practices and ideas are reproduced.

I have argued elsewhere (Iphofen, 1998) that in the field of education, responsibility for learning must be shared: 'Learner responsibility is a joint accomplishment of learner, educator and institution'. In the same way, responsibility for health has to be shared between those who possess the knowledge, skills and access to the finite resources of health which are always in great demand. There is a mutual responsibility between professional and client. It is not enough for the professional to say 'Well, I've told them – now it's up to them to get on with it'. Nor, as demonstrated above, is it always effective to act 'for' the client when they will act in a more sustained and effective way for themselves if they possess the necessary incentives and resources. It is useless to assign responsibility to individuals when they lack the power to act. In the current health care system much of the power is concentrated in the hands of the State and the medical profession. To shift responsibility to the 'patient' without giving them adequate power is to limit their potential for action.

In some respects the professional working to improve public health may resemble a guide on the journey toward health. They may not have travelled some of the paths themselves, but they know the route, having studied it carefully and benefited from the collective experience of their profession. They are then best placed to advise the individual of the most appropriate route. The competent health professional is someone who judges appropriately the timing and the extent of their intervention in the health pursuits of individuals and of communities. The real skill of the public health professional is in achieving the correct balance of responsibility and the most effective employment of their power.

References

Acheson, D. (1998) *Independent Inquiry Into Inequalities in Health*. London: The Stationery Office.

Albrecht, G.L., Fitzpatrick, R. and Scrimshaw, S.C. (eds) (2000) *Handbook of Social Studies in Health and Medicine*. London: Sage.

Atkin, C. and Wallack, L. (1990) *Mass Communication and Public Health*. London: Sage.

Atkinson, P. (1979) The Symbolic Significance of Health Foods. In Turner, M. (ed.) *Nutrition and Lifestyles*. London: Applied Science Publishers.

Batmanghelidj, F. (2000) *Your Body's Many Cries for Water*. Tagman Press.

Bell, D. and Valentine, G. (1997) *Consuming Geographies: We are Where We Eat*. London: Routledge.

Berkman, L.F., Glass, T., Brisette, I. and Seeman, T.E. (2000) From Social Integration to Health: Durkheim in the New Millennium. *Social Science and Medicine*, 51, 843–57.

Brandt, A.M. and Rozin, P. (eds) (1997) *Morality and Health*. London: Routledge.

Brunner, E. and Marmot, M.G. (1999) Social Organisation, Stress and Health. In Marmot, M.G. and Wilkinson, R.G. (eds) *Social Determinants of Health*, Oxford: Oxford University Press.

Bynner, J. and Egerton, M. (2001) *The Wider Benefits of Higher Education*. Institute of Education, University of London (HEFCE and Smith Institute sponsored) Report No. 46.

Cox, P. and Brusseau, P. (1997) *Secret Ingredients*. London: Bantam Books.

Delphy, C. (1979) Sharing the same table: Consumption and the family. In Harris, C. (ed.) *The Sociology of the Family*, Sociological Review Monograph No. 28.

Diamond, H. and Diamond, M. (1985) *Fit for Life*. London: Bantam Books.

Etzioni, A. (1993) *The Spirit of Community* (Rights, Responsibilities and the Communitarian Agenda). New York: Crown.

Foucault, M. (1980) *Power/Knowledge* (Selected interviews and other writings 1972–1977). New York: Pantheon.

Graham, H. (1993) *Hardship and Health in Womens' Lives*. Brighton: Harvester Wheatsheaf.

Gray, A. (ed.) (2001) *World Health and Disease*. Buckingham: Open University Press.

Greenhalgh, T. and Hurwitz, B. (1999) *Narrative Based Medicine*. London: BMJ Books.

House, J.S., Kessler, R.C., Herzoh, A.R., Mero, R.P., Kinney, A.M. and Breslow, M.J. (1990) Age, socioeconomic status and health. *Milbank Quarterly*, 68, 383–411.

Illich, I. (1977) *Limits to Medicine: Medical Nemesis: The Expropriation of Health*. Harmondsworth: Penguin.

Iphofen, R. and Poland, F. (1998) *Sociology in Practice for Health Care Professionals*. London: Macmillan Press – now Palgrave.

Iphofen, R. (1998) Understanding Motives in Learning: Mature Students and Learner Responsibility. In Brown, S., Armstrong, S. and Thompson, G. (eds) *Motivating Students* London: Kogan Page.

Kawachi, I. and Kennedy, B.P. (1997) Health & Social Cohesion: Why Care About Income Inequality? *British Medical Journal*, 314, 1037–40.

Kelner, M. and Wellman, B. (1997) Health care and Consumer Choice: Medical and Alternative Therapies. *Social Science and Medicine*, 45, 2, 203–12.

Kerr, M. and Charles, N. (1986) Servers and Providers: The Distribution of Food Within the Family. *Sociological Review*, 31, 115–57.

Laurance, J. (2001) In Sickness and in Health. *Search*, 34, 35–8.

Link, B.G. and Phelan, J. (1995) Social Conditions as Fundamental Causes of Disease. *Journal of Health and Social Behaviour* (Extra Issue), 80–94.

Lynch, J.W. and Kaplan, G.A. (1997) Understanding How Inequality in the Distribution of Income Affects Health. *Journal of Health Psychology*, 2, 297–314.

Marinella, M.A., Pierson, C. and Chenoweth, C. (1997) The Stethoscope. A Potential Source of Nosocomial Infection? *Archives of Internal Medicine*, 14 April, 157, 7, 786–90.

Marmot, M., Ryff, C.D., Bumpass, L.L., Shipley, M. and Marks, N.F. (1997) Social Inequalities in Health: Next Questions and Converging Evidence. *Social Science and Medicine*, 44, 901–10.

Marmot, M.G. and Wilkinson, R.G. (eds) (1999) *Social Determinants of Health*. Oxford: Oxford University Press.

McDermott, I. and O'Connor, J. (1996) *NLP and Health*. London: Thorsons.

Mennel, S. (1985) *All Manner of Food*. London: Sage.

Mennell, S., Murcott, A. and van Otterloo, A.H. (1992) *The Sociology of Food & Eating*. London: Sage.

Mitchell, R., Shaw, M. and Dorling, D. (2001) *Inequalities in Life and Death: What if Britain were More Equal?* Oxford: The Policy Press.

Robert, S.A. and House, J.A. (2000) Socioeconomic Inequalities in Health: Integrating Individual-, Community-, and Societal-Level Theory and Research. In Albrecht, G.L., Fitzpatrick, R. and Scrimshaw, S.C. (eds) *Handbook of Social Studies in Health and Medicine*. London: Sage.

Sapolsky, R.M. (1994) *Why Zebras Don't Get Ulcers (A Guide to Stress, Stress-Related Diseases, and Coping)*. New York: W.H. Freeman and Co.

Sokolov, R. (1991) *Why We Eat What We Eat*. New York: Summit Books.

Tenner, E. (1996) *Why Things Bite Back (Technology and the Revenge Effect)*. London: Fourth Estate.

Wilkinson, R.G. (1996) *Unhealthy Societies: The Afflictions of Inequality*. London: Routledge.

Williams, D.R. (1990) Socioeconomic Differentials in Health: A Review and Redirection. *Social Psychology Quarterly*, 53, 2, 81–99.

Williams, R. (1983) Concepts of Health: An Analysis of Lay Logic. *Sociology*, 17, 2, 185–205.

3

Health Inequalities: the Black Report and Beyond

ROSS BROCKLEHURST and JOHN COSTELLO

The key points discussed in this chapter include:

- the extent to which key historical events and social changes have influenced public health and social inequalities prior to the publication of the Black Report

- the influence of government reports, reforms and research relating to inequalities in health experiences of different social groups

- how public health initiatives have sought to address social inequalities since the publication of the Black Report findings.

Introduction

Two fundamental assumptions underpin the writing of this chapter. First, as most health practitioners are aware, health inequalities between individuals exist and, second, their underlying causation is rooted in the prevailing socio-economic conditions within society. Many in modern Western society believe that public health is determined by life-style, which, in itself, is influenced by the social and economic conditions encountered by individuals at any given time. Conversely, others would argue that improvements in public health, accurate diagnosis and effective treatment determine individual and community health. Much of the debate about public health and health inequalities, however, is coloured by differences in the way health is defined and understood by health care professionals, policy makers, economists and social policy analysts. Taking this view, Illich (1976) points out that health care is managed by professionals based on the assumption that it is only they who are able to bring about effective changes in health. The history of public health suggests that conceptualisations of health in secondary and primary care is closely associated with power issues between professionals and their clients and the extent to which people are able to-exert a certain amount of control over their own health experiences.

This chapter identifies the key historical events, including social changes that have influenced health and public health from Victorian times up to the publication of the Black Report in 1980. The discussion demonstrates how improvements in public health in Victorian times arose from social change as well as medical innovation. In doing this, the chapter describes and reviews the effect of legislation, reforms and research relating to health inequalities and traces the origins of the debate that inequalities in health have a causal relationship with the underlying social inequalities. Consistent with the themes of this book, it identifies that despite the ability to exercise power to make changes, little change has taken place in the twenty years since the publication of the Black Report in 1980; if anything the gap between the advantaged and disadvantaged in society is getting wider. Consideration is also given to the current relationship between social and health inequalities and how these are being addressed following the publication of the Black Report.

Public Health and Social Change

One of the most prominent landmarks in British history was the impact of the Victorians on a wide range of social, scientific and health developments. The Victorian era demonstrated wide disparity of health care needs between the poor and the wealthy, with huge social inequalities between these two groups.

Victorian experiences of health reflect the prevailing social and economic conditions during a time of industrialisation, invention and discovery. Many factors contributed to the provision of good health that was medically, socially and politically motivated. One of the most significant features of Victorian public health was sanitation, which became a major public health issue of 1850s Britain. During this period in history, two key issues were prominent in preventing ill health. The first became apparent from the writings of Florence Nightingale (1860) who reported that the general level of health of soldiers fighting in the Crimean War was influenced by nutrition. This highlighted the importance of the dietary needs of 'the labouring population'. Second, soldiers, particularly those who were wounded, became susceptible to diseases because of the lack of clean water, the appalling amount of infection and the lack of medicine to treat the sick. Diseases such as cholera, typhoid and TB accounted for almost as many deaths as the war itself.

Against this backdrop of poor nutrition and the spread of disease, public health reforms during the 1850s in Victorian England demonstrate the fact that improvements in sanitation and nutrition made a significant difference to the health of the lower social classes. The Victorian poor had to rely on the benevolence of others and the hope that their social conditions, and subsequently their standard of health, improved. Irrespective of social class, the population of Victorian London in the 1850s suffered from a lack of proper sewerage systems which gave rise to outbreaks of cholera and typhoid. In 1858, the smell of sewerage from the river Thames, referred to as 'the great stink', was so great that it was suggested that Parliament be relocated away from it (Rosen, 1993). It was not until Basiljet introduced and built a series of 82 miles of sewers underneath London that diseases like typhoid were brought under control and many deaths prevented. An example of the relationship between ill health and social conditions was the parlous state of young men conscripted to the First World War who were found to be malnourished and in a poor physical condition. The legacy of the Victorian era was the need for a welfare system to deal with the health needs of the labouring populations of Britain.

The Need for a Welfare State

A number of writers point out that one of the reasons why politicians argued for the need for a national health service was to prevent and control the health of the poorer classes (Abel-Smith, 1964; Titmuss, 1963; Klein, 1998). These examples demonstrate that public health can be affected by social as well as medical innovations such as the use of penicillin during the Second World War. Historically, the relationship between public health and social inequalities, as Richman and Haggart point out in their chapters, was based on a combination of medical discovery, (Abel-Smith, 1964) social change (Klein, 1998) political reforms and public demand (Titmuss, 1963). By taking a historical perspective, we are able to view the synergy between health and social conditions and to discern how changes in both result from social and medical innovations. As the rest of the chapter outlines, to tackle the fundamental problem of individual health it became essential to consider the underlying conditions that help to develop and sustain differences in health experiences.

Health, Social Inequalities and Entitlement

For many poorer members of society, their only substantive asset is their ability to work. Consequently, when they become unable to work (through ill health) they experience deprivation and, in some cases, death. In relation to entitlement and deprivation Davey-Smith (1996) points out that there is nothing new about the recognition that starvation is best seen as a part of 'entitlement failure'. If the poor are not part of the equal distribution of resources such as material goods, adequate housing, sanitation, food and good hygiene, they experience deprivation, hunger and, as a consequence, loss of health.

Within the health service differences of opinion regarding how to reduce the gap between the health experiences of the rich and poor have resulted in broad divisions about how to improve health and provide effective health care. Graham (2000) argues that much modern medicine was based on untested assumptions and that the values of bio-medicine (the seeking of health problems by using scientific biomedical approaches) were unproven, with little analysis of the effectiveness or efficiency of medical care. In order to properly assess the value of medical interventions, doctors should take full account of social inequalities (Graham, 2000).

In particular, McKeown (1976, 1979) highlights the medical 'success' of treating respiratory tuberculosis (TB) (known to many as consumption) and cholera which were major causes of death largely due to people living in overcrowded areas, polluted environments, and to poor water. The recent resurgence of TB in London (see Costello *et al.*) Chapter 4 demonstrated that for a minority of people their social conditions make them vulnerable to the onset of infectious diseases. As Richman highlights in Chapter 1, social changes have made a major impact on the decline of infectious diseases. McKeown (1979) asserts that medicine has had an exaggerated role in curing illness and has led to increased investment in medical approaches and a 'cure-all' ideology. To make a full contribution to health, medicine needs to be concerned with prevention as well as interventions. Highlighting improvements in nutritional status, living conditions, and better health and safety measures, accounts for the population growth. McKeown makes the point that:

> Contrary to what is generally believed, the most fundamental issue confronting medical science is not the solution of one or more of the unsolved biomedical problems, it is the evaluation of two approaches to the control of disease, one through understanding of mechanisms and the other through a knowledge of origins.

To improve public health therefore, there is clearly a need to seriously consider the underlying social inequalities that contribute to the poor health experiences of many people.

The NHS and Health Inequalities

Advances in health care since the formation of the NHS in 1948 have improved the general health of the population measured against a number of criteria, such as increased numbers of acute patients treated and greater use made of emergency services. Poor housing, poverty and lack of health education played an equal if not more important role in determining the health and well-being of the population.

Despite its success, the NHS does not seem to have made a marked difference to the health experiences of those at different poles of the social class system. The Royal Commission on the NHS (Merrison Report) (1979) identified in its findings that the gradient between the health chances of individuals residing throughout all levels of the social class hierarchy had widened, although mortality rates had begun to fall. The report highlighted that although they were living longer, the health of some individuals was poorer due to living with debilitating chronic illness and disability.

The formation of the NHS represented huge potential for benefiting health and had a major impact by providing universal access to health care. Many gained direct access to acute and primary services designed to cure and prevent diseases that previously caused suffering and death for millions of people. The provision of 'free' health care had a radical impact on the numbers of people who were chronically sick for whom illness was a central part of their lives (Klein, 1998).

The poorer members of society also had a two-and-a-half times greater chance of dying before the age of 65, resulting from ill health as well as increased numbers of deaths from accidents at work (Townsend and Davidson, 1982). The varied reasons for this stemmed from a lack of access to those material and social factors that delayed the onset of ill health (discussed by Iphofen). Poverty, deprivation, lack of access to services and limited understanding of the nature and extent of preventative health care services are the principal barriers to good health.

Why Health Inequalities Persist

A huge amount of research has been conducted on why inequalities exist. Evidence from the literature up to the 1990s underpins the belief that individuals who exist in poor socio-economic circumstances are likely to experience poorer health and develop future health-related problems. The evidence overwhelmingly indicates that this is due to material disadvantage. Health inequalities are interrelated with social inequalities, since housing, life-style, income and employment directly impinge on individual health. The relationship between health problems at the begin-ning and end of life indicates that those less advantaged in society who experience ill health in early childhood often develop problems later in life if their material circumstances remain the same. In other words, individuals born into poverty who remain poor for most of their lives tend to experience poor health at the end of their lives. However, Bartley *et al.* (1998) point out that early life experiences do not have the same effect on later health with all people. Evidence suggests that the more affluent are able to avoid by "shrugging off" poor early life health problems. For those born into depri-vation who experience 'social disadvantage' as a way of life, they often face a downward spiral from which they are unable to recover (Kuh and Davey-Smith, 1993). Evidence suggests that lack of income or deprivation are not the only indicators of poor health (Bartley *et al.*, 1998; Wilkinson, 1986). Bartley *et al.* refer to the 'fine grain' to describe different levels of social differentiation in relation to health risks. The authors cite examples of people with their own homes and two cars as having greater life expectancy than other homeowners with one car. This is an interesting, if not unusual, finding and suggests that the evidence in health inequality research is trying to consider different levels of deprivation as the criteria which apply to individual cases. What may be concluded from the research is that, at an individual level, there is an established link between social inequalities and health inequalities with higher material living standards equating with better opportunities for improved health in the future.

The Influence of Social Class and Employment on Health

Traditional social class groupings such as those described by sociologists Wilmot and Young (1960) in the early 1960s may have limited contempo-rary value for estimating the socio-economic status of large numbers of individuals within society. This may be due to a number of reasons. Chiefly that the instrument used to measure and categorise social class positions, that is the Registrar General's social class scale, is a poor indi-cator of social position, as described in detail by Duke and Edgell (1987). Apart from other reasons, they point out that the scale excludes from the analytical process two-thirds of the members of society such as women, retired people, students and the unemployed.

In order for any assessment of social class to be accurate it would be necessary to review occupation as an indicator although, based on the evidence, one has to question the validity of the Registrar General's scale as anything more than a generalisation about social class positions.

Employment as a source of social identity at the beginning of the twenty-first century has become less significant and, as Gortz (1982) iden- tifies, perhaps it is time to say 'farewell to the working class'. Others point out that there may be alternative methods for estimating social class which are more accurate predictors of health outcome and economic posi- tion and which may be more effective measures such as parental social class, education, family income and housing tenure (Crompton, 1993; Graham, 2000). In contemporary times, Graham points out, differences in rates for those at the top and the bottom of the social hierarchy have widened due to an increasing polarisation of material wealth within the United Kingdom's population. In the 1970s less than 1 in 10 of the popula- tion lived in households with incomes below the EU (European Union) poverty line of less than half the average household income after housing costs (Allen, 1999). In almost all areas of scrutiny, including lung cancer, heart disease, accidents and suicide the poor are more susceptible than the rich. In the late 1990s the proportion was 1 in 4 of households living below the EU poverty line and 34 per cent of those with children being particu- larly impoverished (DSS, 1998). A number of studies demonstrate that, although life expectancy has gradually risen over the last century, illness- free periods remain static and appear to show little improvement. The number of people with long-standing illness, Allen (1999) points out, increased from 15 to 22 per cent of the population as a whole. Employment as an indicator of social position will always be important for denoting social status since its absence carries with it a social stigma. Social class positions, however, remain, at least sociologically, an important but prob- lematic issue and little more than an indicator of social stratification.

The Black Report

The Black Report was not the first major work to address differences in health and link these to social inequalities, but it did create a watershed and, since its publication in 1980, there has been a significant increase in publications on the topic.

The findings from the Black Report's working party (Black et al., 1980) are among the most significant evidence on health inequalities ever pub- lished. The working party was established to examine the broader factors influencing health under the direction of Douglas Black (Chief Scientist at the Department of Health and Social Security).

The members of the working party were clear that health inequalities existed but could not agree about the extent to which changes were required to bring about significant improvements. This debate was confounded by problematic issues to do with defining what health is and reaching agreements about accurate measures for poverty. The working party pointed out that:

> We were all agreed that education and preventative measures, specifically directed towards the socially deprived were necessary. But the sociological members of the group [Townsend and Smith] considered that the consequent expenditure should be obtained by diversion from the acute services. On the other hand medical members – and that means both of us [Black and Morris] – felt that the acute services played a vital part in the prevention of chronic disability and could not be further cut back without serious effects on emergency care, on the training of doctors for both hospital work and for family practice and on the length of waiting lists. We spent a lot of time, without real success trying to resolve this matter.

A brief summary of the working party's key conclusions is given in Table 3.1.

The publication of the report was surrounded in controversy and was received by the newly elected Conservative Government in April 1980, although its release (without a press conference) was delayed until August during parliamentary recess. Only 260 duplicated copies of the report were held by the Department of Health and Social Security. The release of the report made shocking reading as it revealed wide disparities in health experiences of people at opposite ends of the social scale. The reasons for these are complex, with no single redeeming factor emerging. What is clear is the role of certain services, such as ante natal and cervical screening, in picking up many potential health problems. The report highlighted the many life-style factors which correlate with social class differences contributing to the reduction of health chances, such as cigarette smoking, workplace accidents and poor housing.

Table 3.1   A brief summary of the key conclusions of the
Black Report's working party

- Despite advances in health care, the general health of the population as a whole had declined
- The evidence supports the link between poverty and increased experiences of ill health
- Certain socio-economic features of society such as poverty and poor access to health care played an equal if not more important role in determining well-being of the population
- The report identified disparities in the use of the NHS by lower social groups that are still prevalent today

The report also provided four main explanations for why people's experiences of health differed and made many recommendations for rectifying the problem of health inequalities. These included changes in NHS provision as well as investing more resources into tackling social inequalities by increasing welfare benefits, lifting people from poverty by tackling unemployment and raising living standards through better housing. The report's recommendations included creating greater access to primary and secondary health care facilities, especially those preventative services, which could delay the development of chronic illness.

The debate that followed the publication of the Black Report polarised the argument along professional and political grounds. The working group itself was split over how resources should be reallocated and how this would lead to health improvements.

The Government's initial response to the Black Report findings, judged by the activities of the time, clearly suggested that the whole area of health and health provision was very sensitive. The then Conservative Secretary of State for Health, Patrick Jenkins, rejected the recommendations, saying that there was no evidence of the effectiveness of the measures outlined in the report.

Explanations for Health Inequalities

The Artefact Explanation

The artefact explanation (Illsley, 1986; Bloor *et al.*, 1987), at its most basic, refutes the idea that health inequalities really exist. Those using artefact theory question the various interpretations of the evidence. The assumptions being made are that there is no correlation between health and social class and that health inequalities are an artefact of the official statistics-gathering process with no direct relationship between them. The detail of the argument is that, as the proportion of those in lower social classes reduces because of a general increase and distribution of the total wealth of the population, there will be a subsequent reduction in health inequalities. The improved health of those ascending the social class scales, including the lower social classes, continues to be exposed to threats to their health chances. Townsend *et al.* (1988) argue that the number of individuals within lower social classes is not reducing at a commensurate rate to sustain this argument. In addition, they point out that the number of individuals who suffer the consequences of poor health apply to a larger cross-section of the working population, more than those who occupy lower positions on the social class scale. The processes involved in social class categorisation play a part in the structure of the artefact. Illsley (1986) and Bloor *et al.* (1987) suggest that the Registrar General's classification created a hundred years ago is no longer relevant and its operation exaggerates health differences. These authors point out that the classification and nature of occupations has changed considerably over time. Simultaneously, however, the social context and the influences on individual and community health have not remained constant over time. Whitehead (1987) asserts that the elimination of time effects on occupational class data show that none of the results alters the overall picture to any great extent. The artefact explanation does not provide any substantive evidence that differences between the health of groups are not related to socio-class groupings.

Studies undertaken since the publication of the Black Report findings suggest that, whatever measure of social difference is applied, health inequalities are demonstrated between those at the top and bottom of the social class scale. The preoccupation with social class and its usefulness detracts from the main argument. Levels of material wealth negatively influence the health of poorer members of society with greater wealth and economic security having a positive effect on health experiences.

Natural/Social Selection Explanation

The theoretical framework underpinning the natural and social selection explanation is that a person's position in the occupational class system is determined by their physical and mental health. Crudely put, this theory may be seen as 'the survival of the fittest', with the weakest suffering greater hardship. In this sense health is defined as physical and mental strength. When a person's health deteriorates, they may lose their job and move down the social class hierarchy, hence the 'survival of the fittest', the key element being that a person's prior health status determines their social position. The basic premise of the natural selection argument is based on the assumption that individuals who occupy superior positions in society tend to be the most healthy in the population. Those who occupy positions within assumedly subordinate positions (social classes 4 and 5) are, by definition, the weakest and less healthy. Using this theory, physical weakness therefore determines lower social position with less potential for social reward or material wealth. The assumption being made is that material surroundings or wealth play no part in predicting the possibility of the individual being exposed to a higher future mortality. Furthermore, by adopting the essential elements of this model, it may be argued that ill health can lead to unemployment as opposed to unemployment leading to poor health (Blane *et al.*, 1993).

Materialist Theory

This theory suggests that differences in material wealth account for health differences and that those who experience most deprivation, such as poor housing and low income, experience greater health inequalities. An example of this is the social experiences of childhood poverty affecting the ability of children to reach their fullest health potential (Whitehead, 1987). Power (1991) identifies the confusion about the effects of childhood deprivation and that the effects of deprivation in childhood and experiences such as teenage pregnancy can also shape experiences in adult life. In adulthood, becoming sick often means becoming unable to develop materially or economically (Blackburn, 1991). However, being sick in itself is not understood enough for us to explain health differentials between social classes. Golblatt (1990) notes that changes in individual social class positions during middle age have no discernible effect on the mortality rate of the individual. The notion of materialism argues that if physical strength determines social position then, as health deterioration occurs, individual ability to work declines and, when unable to work, social mobility is reduced. In this way, the link between social class categorisation and health becomes redefined.

Cultural and Behaviour Explanation

Cultural/behavioural explanations for health inequalities point out that class differences in terms of beliefs about health, health behaviour and life-style are responsible for health and social conditions and circumstances play a part in being healthy. This issue, taken up previously in Ron Iphofen's chapter, looks at the influence of behaviour, beliefs, customs and traditions on health and well-being. As Iphofen points out, most people lighting a cigarette, eating junk food or 'being a couch potato' are not attempting to reproduce patterns of health inequality. What we know from research is that people who tend to adopt an unhealthy life-style tend to come from poorer social groups. An example of this in relation to manual workers equates good health with the absence of symptoms and good fortune (Field, 1995).

The theoretical framework underpinning cultural/behavioural explanations highlights the importance of social conditions and circumstances in individual health and that life-style is responsible in some way for health. Inequalities in health, according to this theory, stem from those most disadvantaged in society adopting more dangerous, risk-orientated life-styles such as smoking, drinking to excess and having poor diets which may have their origins in social class attitudes. This is compared to the less risk-centred life-style of the most advantaged members of society. Cultural/behavioural explanations point to the importance of the environment and place emphasis upon the unhealthy environments of both domestic and work-related domains of life such as poor housing, living in deprived areas and working in high-risk occupations such as the building industry. Evidence suggests that children from disadvantaged families are at more risk from childhood accidents resulting from their environment (Blaxter, 1990). Blane (1985) points out that those using this type of explanation tend to separate out behaviour from the social context in which it takes place. The higher percentage of male and female cigarette smokers in lower social classes seems to support this view, as fewer adult smokers by comparison are located in higher social groups (ONS, 1998). The questions we perhaps need to ask are about why those in the most disadvantaged groups seem least able to adopt healthier life-styles.

Beyond the Black Report

The most significant response made to the findings of the Black Report was the Acheson Report, published in 1998, which was commissioned by the incoming Labour Government to review the evidence available on health inequalities with the aim of informing and identifying future policy development. The report recognised the findings of the Black Report as well as being responsive to the limited implementation of many of its findings. The report may be seen as a response to the Government's recognition that the country was divided by social class, gender and ethnicity and that these inequalities had been worsening for twenty years. The recommendations made by the Acheson Committee amounted to a review of the Black Report findings but, unlike its predecessor, contained no reference to cost of health services. Instead, the Acheson Report (1998) highlighted the need for increased prioritisation of family health services, especially for those with children. The report made specific recommendations that steps be taken to reduce income inequalities and improve living standards of poorer households. The need for this issue to be highlighted is a sad indictment of the failure of Government to make a positive response to the findings of the Black Report less than twenty years earlier, as well as an alarming reflection on the nation's health. It seems absurd to think that a highly industrialised, prosperous nation such as Britain, where the 50 richest people have a net wealth of £34 billion, should have people dying because they do not properly use available health services. The report's recommendations made a statement expressing commitment to young children and their mothers, disabled people and measures concerned with prevention. The specific recommendations relating to children and mothers are illustrated in Table 3.2.

The report referred to actions that may be taken to improve the care of the elderly and disabled in the community and identified national health goals to be made transparent following debate and consultation. The report highlighted measures to be taken to encourage desirable changes in individual life-styles relating to diet, exercise, smoking and drinking and the provision of a counselling service in all health districts to help people to reduce cigarette smoking. Table 3.3 outlines the key areas relating to the enlargement of a programme of health education directly supported by Government.

A wide-ranging set of recommendations was made to constrain tobacco sponsorship, advertising and consumption with a view to phasing out

Table 3.2   Specific health and welfare measures for mothers
and pre-school children

- Introduction of free milk to the first-born and to children from large families (Chapter 8)
- Reviews of ante-natal and child health provision and accessibility in order to increase uptake in the early months of pregnancy
- Savings made from the reduction in the school population to be redirected into the provision of new services for the under-5s
- School health care to be integrated into generic community medical services and health screening and surveillance in areas of special need to be intensified
- Abolition of child poverty as a priority for the 1980s
- Action to be taken to reduce accidents to children

Table 3.3   Key areas of the Acheson Report relating to
health education

- Health education in schools should be the joint responsibility of LEAs and health authorities
- Measures to reduce cigarette smoking, including the phasing out of all advertising
- Government to fund and finance a special health and social development programme in a small number of selected areas, at an estimated cost of £30 million
- The introduction of a comprehensive disablement allowance for all introduced by stages

the production of harmful tobacco products (Acheson Report, 1998, Chapter 8:162).

The report's authors went on to state that their recommendations were set in the belief that they had focused on those factors that correlated with a degree of health inequality.

Health Divide Revisited

The legacy of the Black Report has had a powerful impact on public health thinking partly due to the initial attempts to suppress the findings. Whitehead (1987) co-edited the paperback version of the Black Report in 1982 with Townsend and Davidson and was a major standard bearer for the Black Report findings. Her work focused on the differences in health and social inequalities, concentrating on differential resources as well as updating and reinforcing the Black Report findings. Essentially, Whitehead focused much attention on differences between different parts of the country in what is simplistically referred to as the north–south divide, with Scotland having some of the worst health profiles. Scotland in terms of health spending has reached the EEC average of 8 per cent of GNP because of a favourable subsidy formula by Westminister. This high-lights the view that resources need not be a major factor in the health debate. Whitehead's work received greater organisational publicity than the Black Report, much to the Government's annoyance. The health divide drew attention to regional differences and class divisions, attracting criti-cism from government supporters that it had a Marxist bias. Whitehead focused much attention on class divisions and reliance on the Registrar General's classification which, in itself, limited the visibility of women since social class (according to the Registrar's scale) was determined by male occupation. Whitehead's thesis highlighted differences in living con-ditions between regions in the north and south but failed to acknowledge fundamental social issues such as changing family patterns, increased numbers of women in the labour market, increased divorced and one-parent families (Dennis and Erdos, 1995; Morgan, 1995).

The notion of inequality has always been problematic from an ideologi-cal perspective. The idea of 'classless societies' is considered by many to have become a myth, with social engineering to achieve this aim being extremely difficult if not impossible. Poverty, specifically, has proved to be very problematic, not least in terms of definition. In the nineteenth century the Rowntree (1901) studies of York considered the concept of 'absolute poverty' to involve the required number of calories and minimum wage needed for life support. Under the influence of Townsend (1973), poverty levels were considered to be *relative* to levels of spending and based on family dietary patterns and the amount of material consumption. Measurement of poverty as relative or absolute reveal interesting comparative features, as Gordon *et al.* (2000) found in their study of adult poverty in Britain. Men were generally more likely than women to specify some items and activities as essential, such as 'having a small amount of money to spend on yourself', being able to go to the pub and having new, not second-hand, clothes. In political terms there are many who fear that New Labour's crusade to eliminate poverty is doomed (see Costello, Chapter 8 for further discussion). In terms of dealing effectively with poverty and inequalities, evidence from other countries, such as Japan and Sweden, suggests that societies that have a convergence of income distribution and further redistribution of wealth have much lower levels of health inequality. Spicker (2002) and Startup (2002) highlight how countries with some of the best health profiles that also use health rationing are much more able to help to remedy major differences in access to, and take-up of, health resources. As the evidence demonstrates, most countries have health divides and in many cases differences within individual regions as a result of varying levels of poverty. It would seem therefore that one way forward in reducing health divides is to look closely at the causes of poverty and how these perpetuate health and social inequality.

Do Health and Social Inequalities Still Exist?

In looking beyond the Black Report, there is clear evidence that social inequalities relate to and underpin health inequalities today and in some cases there is evidence that the gap between social classes in terms of health experiences is widening (Blane *et al.*, 1993). Despite the many criticisms of social class as an effective way of measuring social divisions (Bloor *et al.*, 1987), it is clear that Britain remains largely divided by class. Contemporary research findings reinforce the view that health inequalities cannot easily be explained away by artefact and social selection theories. Much more expansion is needed of the materialist and cultural theories in order to develop a more accurate picture of their cogency as explanations. The debate concerning health inequalities has moved on considerably taking account of the huge changes and social developments that have taken place in British society since the Black Report was published (see, for example, Costello *et al.*'s discussion of globalisation) in the next chapter which have impacted on the structure of society and its response to the need for social reform. One of the developments was the findings from the Office of National Statistics Longitudinal study (LS) (Fox and Golblatt, 1982) which indicated that mortality differences between the highest and lowest social classes had widened between 1961 and 1971. An interesting methodological feature of this research was the confirmation that the evidence of health inequalities was not due to statistical bias and refutes the artefact theory. The four explanations given for health inequalities need to be modified on the basis of findings from contemporary research which takes into account the many social changes that have taken place in the last twenty years.

Why Do Inequalities in Health Persist?

Three areas of concern become the focus of this discussion which makes the point that not only do health inequalities continue to exist but also the reasons why are becoming more clear as a result of social changes and research. First, the notion of life-style and its effects on health, second, the impact of sustained social inequality on a person's mental health and, third, the effects of powerful groups limiting individual opportunities for health. Many of the indirect/direct causes of death across social class categorisations relate to what may be called 'diseases of affluence' such as eating, drinking and smoking. In relation to life-style it is clear, as Iphofen points out in Chapter 2 that it is futile to give responsibility to individuals when they lack the power to act. In other words, if an individual has a poor diet and a so-called 'bad life-style' likely to make their health worse, there is little point in telling them that the best thing they can do is to change their habits. They are just as likely to ask what the second best thing is as they cannot do the first. Health care professionals need to be able to assess their clients and empower them to make the necessary changes themselves or advocate on their behalf (see Haggart, Chapter 9). Providing responsibility to the client without giving them the necessary power is likely to frustrate them and cause them to feel more powerless. As Bartley *et al.* (1998) point out, it is important to consider that the causes of inequality are not just about the impact of the social environment. Hence, the social selection theory is limited in its belief that the weakest in society will always suffer greater deprivation.

The effects of sustained inequalities over a long period on the patient's physical condition are well known. Less well known is the impact of material deprivation on mental health. Within the chapter, the argument has been made that material deprivation accounts for much individual suffering. When this occurs over a lifetime, the effects on the individual in terms of morbidity and mortality are well known, but that individual's ability to sustain themselves and their families is limited. Their coping mechanisms often derive from social support obtained from family and friends.

A number of authors however, point out that as families become impoverished, families as social groups can have adverse psychological effects
on individual members, making it more difficult for families to maintain
social bonds and maintain the self-esteem of individual members
(Wilkinson and Kawachi, 1998; Graham, 1999). Without such social integration, the normal rules of coping may well deteriorate and the individual may become aggressive in order to maintain their sense of social
honour. It may be argued that those who live in a society where there are
marked differences in income may experience hostility and a need to protect themselves from those experiencing the effects of deprivation
(Hutton, 1996).

Finally, as globalisation and capitalism expands, the importance of
employment in terms of protecting individuals and communities becomes
clear. The increasing power of technology and the impact of globalisation
(see Costello *et al.*'s chapter) mean that those lower down the social scale
are more likely to find themselves socially excluded as a result of corpo-
rations 'shedding' the workforce, resulting in higher unemployment. This
is surely not about the weakness of the worker but about power and the
need for capitalism to achieve its aim of securing profit at the expense of
creating surplus workforce with little thought to the consequences.

Conclusion

The issues around health inequalities have been on the health policy
agenda for many years. The arguments pervade and are supported by the
philosophical, often political and, moreover, the professional doctrine of
health and social welfare reformers. At the centre of these discussions is the
issue of cost and whether the Government of the day is prepared to commit itself to meeting these costs and to address issues relating to health
inequality. This chapter has reviewed the findings of the Black Report and
those of the Acheson Report, incorporating an evaluation of the various
explanations for health inequality. The clear indications are that social
inequalities are interconnected with health problems. The varying material
and cultural explanations strongly indicate that, for the disadvantaged, the
adoption of unhealthy life-styles may be seen more usefully as a means of
coping with the deprivation. The backdrop of current social inequalities is
the increasing potential for unemployment and the link between material
loss and social exclusion. The need to generate greater understanding of
the impact of deprivation and the challenge to find links between unhealthy
life-style and ill health needs to be taken up. The explanations for health
inequalities have been explored by many reviewers, and from the more

basic explanations derive an ever-more complex series of sub-textual explanations. It is refreshing that contemporary authors are embarking on studies that place the individual at the centre of their studies. This removes the need to use variables that cannot be fixed over time or across differing communities, such as class-based explanations. The use of small-scale qualitative studies is an attempt to allow researchers access to the lives of those who are at risk of having their lives damaged or curtailed by the operation of health inequality. By understanding the lives and experiences of these groups it may be possible to determine health and social policy options that will address these serious issues. It cannot be acceptable for all of us in this society to allow such a variation in health-related experience of individual members. It is unacceptable that there are simple measures that can be adopted that may reduce the eventual need to commit huge resources to treating the consequences of health and social inequality as opposed to preventing it. In looking beyond the recommendations of the Black Report, it is interesting to see how these initiatives are able to influence social welfare and health policy and change future directives aimed at closing the gap in health inequalities.

References

Abel-Smith, B. (1964) *The Hospitals of England and Wales 1800–1948*. Cambridge, MA: Harvard University Press.

Acheson, D. (1998) *Independent Enquiry into Inequalities in Health*. London: Stationery Office.

Allen, D. (1999) Back in the Black. *Community Practitioner*, 72, 2.

Bartley, M., Blane, D. and Davey-Smith, G.D. (1998) Introduction: beyond the Black Report. *Sociology of Health and Illness*, 20, 5, 563–77.

Black, D., Morris, J., Smith, C. and Townsend, P. (1980) *Inequalities in Health: report of a Working Party*. London: Department of Health and Social Security.

Blackburn, C. (1991) *Poverty and Health*. Milton Keynes: Open University Press.

Blane, D. (1985) An Assessment of the Black Report's Explanations of Health Inequalities. *Sociology of Health and Illness*, 7, 423–45.

Blane, D., Davey-Smith, G. and Bartley, M. (1993) Social Selection: What Does it Contribute to Social Class Differences in Health? *Sociology of Health and Illness*, 15, 1.

Blaxter, M. (1990) *Health and Life-styles*. London: Routledge.

Bloor, M., Samphier, M. and Prior, L. (1987) Artefact explanations of Inequalities Health: an Assessment of Evidence. *Sociology of Health and Illness*, 9, 231–64.

Crompton, R. (1993) *Class and Stratification*. Cambridge: Polity Press.

Davey-Smith, G. (1996) Income inequality and mortality – why they are related – income inequality goes hand in hand with under investment in human resources. *British Medical Journal*, 312, 987–8.

Dennis, N. and Erdos, G. (1995) *Families Without Fatherhood*. London: Institute for the studies of civil society.

DoH (Department of Health) (1999) *Saving Lives Our Healthier Nation*. London: HMSO.

DSS (Department of Social Security) (1998) *Households Below Average Income 1979 to 1996/7*. London: HMSO.

Duke, V. and Edgell, S. (1987) The operationalization of class in British sociology. *British Journal of Sociology*, 38, 445–63.

Field, D. (1995) Social definitions of health and Illness. In Field, D. and Taylor, S. (eds) *Sociology of Health and Health Care*. London: Blackwell.

Fox, A.J. and Golblatt, P. (1982) *Socio-demographic Differentials in Mortality: The OPCS Longitudinal Study*. London: HMSO.

Golblatt, P. (1990) Mortality and alternative social classifications. In Golblatt, P. (ed.) *Longitudinal Study: Mortality and Social Organisation*. London: HMSO.

Gordon, D., Adelman, L., Ashworth, K., Bradshaw, J., Levitas, R., Middleton, S., Pantazis, C., Patsios, D., Payne, S., Townsend, P. and Williams, J. (2000) *Poverty and Social Exclusion (PSE) in Britain*. York: Joseph Rowntree Foundation.

Graham, H. (1999) Inequalities in health: patterns, pathways and policy. *Community Practitioner*, 72, 2.

Graham, H. (2000) The Challenge of Heath Inequalities. In Graham, H. (ed.) *Understanding Health Inequalities*. Buckingham: Open University Press.

Gortz, A. (1982) *Farewell to the Working Class*. London: Pluto.

Hutton, W. (1996) *The State We're In*. London: Jonathan Cape.

Illich, I. (1976) *Medical Nemesis – The Expropriation of Health*. London: Marion Boyars.

Illsley, R. (1986) Occupational Class Selection and the Production of Inequalities in Health. *Quarterly Journal of Social Affairs*, 2, 2, 151–60.

Klein, R. (1998) *The New Politics of the NHS* (3rd edn). London: Longman.

Kuh, D. and Davey-Smith, G. (1993) When is mortality risk determined? Historical insights into a current debate. *Social History of Medicine*, 6, 101–23.

Merrison Report (1979) Royal Commission on the NHS report. Cmnd 7615, London: HMSO.

McKeown, T. (1976) *The Modern Rise of Population*. London: Edward Arnold.

McKeown, T. (1979) *The Role of Medicine*. Oxford: Basil Blackwell.

Morgan, P. (1995) *Farewell to the Family: Public Policy and Family Breakdown in Britain and the USA*. London: IEA health and welfare unit.

Nightingale, F. (1860) *Notes on Nursing: What is is and What it is Not*. London: Harrison.

ONS (Office for National Statistics) (1998) *Living in Britain; Results from the 1996 General Household Survey*. London: The Stationery Office.

ONS (Office for National Statistics) (2002) *Life Expectancy by Region*. London: The Stationery Office.

Power, C. (1991) Social and Economic Background and Class Inequalities in Health Among Young Adults. *Social Science and Medicine*, 32, 411–17.

Rosen, G. (1993) *A History of Public Health*. Baltimore: John Hopkins University Press.

Rowntree, B.S. (1901) *Poverty: a Study of Town Life*. London: Macmillan, now Palgrave.

Spicker, R. (2002) *Poverty and the Welfare State: Dispelling the Myths*. London: Social Market Foundation.

Startup, T. (2002) *Poor Measures*. London: Social Market Foundation.

Titmuss, R. (1963) *Essays on the Welfare State*. London: George Allen & Unwin.

Townsend, P. (1973) Poverty as relative deprivation. In Wedderburn, D. (ed.) *Poverty, Inequality and the Class Structure*. Cambridge, UK: Cambridge University Press.

Townsend, P. and Davidson, N. (1982) *Inequalities in Health: the Black Report*. London: Penguin Books.

Townsend, P., Davidson, N. and Whitehead, M. (1988) *Inequalities in Health: the Black Report*. London: Penguin Books.

Whitehead, M. (1987) *The Health Divide: Inequalities in Health in the 1980s*. London: Health Education Council.

Wilkinson, R.G. (1986) Income and mortality. In Wilkinson, R.G. (ed.) *Class and Health: Research and Longitudinal Data*. London: Tavistock.

Wilkinson, R.G. and Kawachi, I. (1998) *Sociology of Health and Illness*, 20, 5, 563–77.

Wilmot, P. and Young, M. (1960) *Family and Class in a London Suburb*. London: Routledge and Kegan Paul.

Part II

Public Health and Control: Social Responsibility for the Promotion of Health

Part II (Chapters 4, 5 and 6) examines the need for public health services and their utilisation by vulnerable groups, including those from diverse communities (Chapter 4). This chapter looks at the experiences of ethnic minority groups in Britain and focuses on the Chinese community as an illustration of how traditional values and beliefs about health can co-exist within the ideology of Western medicine. Chapter 5 looks at vulnerable social groups in society and, using case study material, illustrates how vulnerability can be created by social forces that seek to marginalise certain members of society. This chapter examines the way in which powerful institutions influence individual vulnerability and perpetuates the process of marginalisation which is an issue explored in detail in subsequent chapters. Chapter 6 examines the way media constructions of health influence, limit and circumscribe our thinking about healthy lifestyles and offers a critique of the way in which health is promoted and controlled by powerful media forces, using television as an exemplar. The chapter considers the pervasive influence of the media on individuals, emphasising the lack of individual power to bring about change in health behaviour.

4

Public Health Issues in Diverse Ethnic Groups

JOHN COSTELLO, JOEL RICHMAN and LOUISE WONG

The key points discussed in this chapter include:

- the issues of multiculturalism in Britain in relation to the public health needs of people from diverse communities
- social influences which impact on multiculturalism and globalisation in diverse communities
- the impact of cultural identity on access to health care, highlighting a need for greater levels of cultural sensitivity in provision of services.

Introduction

The public health needs of many people from so-called 'ethnic minority' groups are under-researched and poorly appreciated. Within contemporary Britain there is evidence of ethnocentricity, a tendency to view one's own cultural identity as the centre of everything, the standard against which all others are judged. In all areas of public life, and notably health care, we see evidence of health inequalities experienced by those who do not share the same cultural beliefs as the resident majority in Britain. As Acheson (1988) has pointed out, public health may be seen as both the science and the art of preventing disease, but it is also concerned with prolonging and promoting life and improving the health of all individuals and communities through the organised efforts of society. The focus of the 'new public health' (Peterson and Lupton, 1996) places population and environment centre-stage and highlights the need to look at the impact of globalisation, multiculturalism and the need for service providers to create and maintain greater cultural sensitivity towards those from diverse communities.

This chapter sets out to critically examine three major aspects of social life that effect the public health of people from ethnic minorities: multiculturalism, globalisation and the need for greater cultural sensitivity or cultural competence. The first is examined and clarified by setting out a number of ideas that provide a micro-sociology of social life by examining how 'open and closed' social networking can enable cultural groups to co-exist within wider society. This chapter sets out the argument that multiculturalism, in terms of the assimilation of all cultures blending into one form of 'Britishness', is problematic. The notion of assimilation, the drawing in of other cultural groups to adapt to their new cultural identity, ignores the power of culture and the need for individuals to be themselves and 'own' their identity. The idea that society shares a common set of values and beliefs about life in general and health in particular is encouraged by globalisation which is examined as a major force in shaping health and attitudes towards illness.

Multiculturalism and globalisation form central planks of the chapter which looks at the impact that both of these ideas have on the provision of public health for people from mixed cultures living in one society. The chapter challenges the assertion made by politicians in Britain that people from other cultures should adapt and accommodate themselves to the dominant British culture. Instead of blaming those from other cultures for not 'fitting into' our culture, we should look at our ability to understand the beliefs, values and attitudes of other cultural groups, or cultural competence, and ask why we in Britain are unable to accommodate other cultures without prejudice and discrimination. By illustrating the way of life of Chinese people, living in Manchester, who practice traditional Chinese medicine, the chapter sets out to examine the values, beliefs and attitudes which make up traditional Chinese culture. The chapter concludes by arguing for the need for cultural sensitivity and for greater understanding of the lay beliefs of other cultures. This, the authors believe, will enable health professionals and policy makers to celebrate the diversity of other cultures without resorting to the need to force ethnic groups to conform to a culture which is both alien and unsympathetic to the value of other cultural experiences.

Ethnic Minorities

The term 'ethnic minorities' is utilised in the chapter because it has been widely adopted in policy discussions in the UK to refer to members of groups who have classified themselves in terms of one of the UK census categories other than 'white'. It is acknowledged that this term is ambiguous, but it is used to stimulate communication and wider debate on the issues. For a more focused view on this point see Gerrish (2000).

All the major cities in the UK have high numbers of ethnic minorities which began to develop centuries ago although the 1950s saw a resurgence. The diversity of ethnic groups makes it extremely difficult to generalise about any one group, although certain characteristics such as high unemployment and poor living standards are recurring features in the majority.

Amin and Oppenheim (1992:63) point out that 'To be born into an ethnic minority in Britain – particularly … whose origins are in Bangledesh, Caribbean or Pakistan – is to face a higher risk of leading a life marked by low income, repeated unemployment, poor health and housing … than someone who is white'. Ethnic minority groups are those perceived to share different cultural norms (identities) from those of the majority group in a multicultural society. This implies that the term 'ethnic minority' is constructed from the social relations that exist between those who are in the ethnic majority. Ethnicity and the linked notion of multiculturalism impinge heavily on public health and social welfare. To date there are few clear indications of just how many different ethnic communities abide in Britain, the most ethnically mixed country in Europe (Lister, 2001). An ethnic group may be seen as a group of people sharing a cultural identity which arises from a collective sense of history and in some cases language. Ethnicity is an imprecise and problematic term used to refer more often to cultural identity and is very distinct from race. Traditional research using the broad term 'Asian' failed to capture some of the complexity of different cultural responses to health and illness. According to Jary and Jary (2000) ethnic groups 'possess their own sense of culture, customs, beliefs and social norms'. The inter-cultural contact between different groups has an ancient tradition and the exchange of ideas and sharing between groups is as old as history itself. The early anthropologists were fascinated by other cultures and became preoccupied with studying the customs, beliefs and practices of other cultures, spending many years living and working with tribal communities, for example, Evans-Pritchard and Malinowski.

Culture and Health

Much research into health and culture identified differences in infant mortality, identifying in particular that the children of mothers from Bangladesh had lower levels of infant mortality than those born in Britain. The children of these mothers born in Britain showed higher infant mortality levels largely because they failed to 'take up' antenatal services. Afro-Caribbeans experience much more sickle cell disease and have mortalities from TB, hypertension, cardiovascular disease, diabetes and liver cancer. There is also evidence of higher levels of mental illness among Afro-Caribbean people living in Britain, particularly schizophrenia. Many of the diseases, such as sickle cell disease, could be prevented if sufficient screening was available (Lister, 2000). Southern Asian people from India also experience a greater incidence of rickets and osteomalacia, and eye conditions such as glaucoma. The spread of such disease among ethnic groups reflects the lack of attention by Western medicine to the needs of marginalised groups. Also, as Lister (2000) points out, the dominance of Western culture and its failure to provide 'affordable solutions' to medical problems such as AIDS has led to a reappraisal of the value of traditional healers and methods because of the undermining of local cultures. The problem is how to support the positive initiatives of such traditions while avoiding the negative features such as female genital mutilation.

Less emphasis is placed on the psychological problems of ethnic minority groups, many of whom following immigration to the UK experience a huge amount of change and have to make necessary adaptations to new conditions. These can give rise to severe psychological trauma or culture shock, the greater the change or the greater the resistance (to their arrival) experienced from the dominant culture, the higher the incidence of mental ill health (Furnham and Bochner, 1990). This may account for why so many people from ethnic groups receive treatment for mental illness (Owusu-Bempah and Howitt, 2000).

Mental ill health and the psychological implications of living in a multicultural society, such as cultural isolation or cultural suffering, are identified by Furnham and Bochner (1990) and described as requiring considerable adjustment if they are not to become an inevitable health problem. Some psychological problems, such as homesickness and loneliness, are inevitable, although others, such as financial stress, lack of employment and ethnocentricity (focus on the values of the dominant cultural group), are avoidable. Table 4.1 sets out the key problems arising from African students studying in Britain.

The institutions they are associated with, such as schools and universities, deal with the health problems of many transient groups such as students from other cultures. The range of health problems such as non-specific physical problems such as tiredness, social withdrawal and passivity may be similar to the problems experienced by asylum seekers in the UK. The lacklustre image and dishevelled appearance may mask a sense of isolation, loneliness and depression. Ward's (1967) study of foreign students in the USA highlighted these symptoms and labelled them 'foreign student syndrome'. He regarded them as suffering from a wide range of non-specific problems related to the suffering from culture shock. One of the most effective ways of surviving the traumas associated with

Table 4.1 Common causes of psychological stress for
African students studying in Britain

Inevitable problems	
British peculiarities	Sexual problems
Racial discrimination	Career – choice restrictions
Accommodation difficulties	Study method discrepancies
Separation reactions	Dietary difficulties
Age determined problems	Personality problems
Language and adjustment	British climate

Source: Zwingmann and Gunn (1983) *Uprooting and health: psychological problems of students from abroad*, Geneva, World Health Organisation, Division of Mental Health.

adapting in a foreign culture is to remain with others who share your experiences and to form associations to protect and offer self-supportive strategies. The question arises then as to how ethnic minorities exist and develop as groups in Britain and in particular how families manage their adaptation to a new culture.

Closed and Open Networks

One of the interesting features of diverse ethnic groups in the UK is their cohesiveness and ability to self-organise despite many of the negative impediments previously discussed. One way of analysing the social organisation of different groups is by studying the networking patterns or social relationships and how many groups conduct and manage themselves through their kinship connections (Richman, 1987). Networking involves examining and identifying relationships and patterns of activity, a trait of social anthropologists. Two types of network structures may be identified, closed and open, which are not isolated features of ethnic groups but emerge from the work of anthropologists and sociologists in the 1950s and 1960s when describing traditional working-class communities (Wilmot and Young, 1960; Gluckman, 1964; Bott, 1971).

Closed networks are those whereby the internal organisation of the family/group is kept within the small circle of family members. Radcliff-Brown (1956) discusses the linkages, patterns and interactional processes of closed networks, highlighting how information about such things as emotional issues, financial problems, illness or relationship matters are not discussed outside the family and advice is not sought in closed networks.

A feature of such closed networks was their cohesiveness and absence of marital breakdown.

Open networks allow for transmission of information and for outside involvement, and are less secretive in terms of their openness to outsiders. In terms of ethnic minority families they invite expert opinion such as doctors and health care workers to advise on how best to manage their affairs. These networks were very instrumental in family life. The Seebohm Report (1968) into the reorganisation of social work in the 1960s highlighted the importance of family networks. The report emphasised how the notion of community implies the existence of networks of reciprocal relationships which, among other things, provided support and basic aid for those experiencing the network. Networks in the context of social work are seen as supportive structures. Richman (1987) points out the existence of networks when examining differential infant mortality, highlighting how low infant mortality rates among working class women could be attributed to family networks which had been in place for many years. In such families women as mothers and mothers-in-law were extremely influential as opinion leaders in terms of childbirth. Working-class women never attended the antenatal clinic, their experts on childbirth were their mothers-in-law with whom many women lived during the early years of their marriage. Newcomers to the area with no closed networks or ties became connected to the medical network system.

Applying this approach to ethnic minority groups, Richman (1987) argues that a feature of many ethnic groups is that they adopt a closed network. This enables the members to protect themselves from outside scrutiny and enables them to survive and develop without harm to their members. The disadvantages are that if family members wish to leave, rebel or challenge the authority of the group, sanctions may be imposed. Many South Asian ethnic groups demonstrate patriarchal structures with men often being instrumental in decision making on behalf of women. Arranged marriages and proximity of housing and attendance at family rituals tend to be proscribed. From the health perspective, lay beliefs about solutions to health problems may be based on the underlying values of the family transmitted through many generations and passed from mother to mother, possibly originating in traditional beliefs about witchcraft.

The Ethnic Minority Experience of Living in Britain

What we know about the social life of people from so-called ethnic minority groups is that their health experiences are often poor (see Brocklehurst and Costello's chapter) and they often experience various forms of discrimination in the form of racism, especially in the workplace. Nehru (1936) provides a historical perspective that by and large remains in evidence today: 'I have become a queer mixture of the East and the West, out of place everywhere, at home nowhere ... I am a stranger and alien in the West. I cannot be of it. But in my own country also, sometimes, I have an exile's feelings.'

Howitt and Owusu-Bempah (1999) indicate that the research evidence on cultural stereotypes demonstrates how professionals such as doctors and psychologists through their interventions display prejudice. The authors cite limited employment opportunities and incorrect psychiatric labelling as major areas where decisions about members of ethnic groups often result in negative stereotyping as a result of assumptions made about culture and religion. Examples include Sikhs being refused work because they refuse to take off their turbans (Bourne *et al.*, 1994). Children from diverse communities also experience prejudice by being refused admission to schools on the basis that they violate dress codes or, for young men, refusing to shave off their beards leads to exclusion from school (Bourne, 1994:29). Mahoney (1988) points out that the notion of multiculturalism in relation to children's experience of education highlights how Britain has a long way to go in coming to terms with what to do about meeting and appreciating the diverse needs of so many who experience state education as a form of oppression. Owusu-Bempah and Howitt (2000) refer to this type of prejudice as 'behavioural apartheid'. Further evidence suggests that certain cultural groups are discriminated against through the lack of health service provision such as the limited amount of screening facilities throughout the country for sickle cell anaemia, a major problem with members of Afro-Caribbean communities (Field and Taylor, 1995). It may be argued therefore that on the basis of the evidence, life in contemporary Britain for many ethnic minorities is difficult due to the alienating effects of living in a different culture but also adapting to change when there is a feeling of animosity shown by certain members of the dominant culture. The accounts of ethnic minority 'user groups' (Gerrish *et al.*, 1996) recalling their hospital experiences indicate the extent to which language plays a major part in helping people feel included in the health care system. Greater use of interpreters could also have helped many of the Somali, Chinese and Gujarati patients have more positive hospital experiences, as well as a higher standard of food! Another illustration of negative attitudes towards ethnic groups is the way in which asylum seekers are being treated today and the political strategies used to 'process' these newcomers by isolating them in quasi-prison environments, reflects a society that is indifferent and at times hostile to the idea of developing a positive multicultural society.

Ethnicity and Race

Today evidence of tension between different ethnic groups evinced through race riots and forms of racism in many public services, such as the police, draws attention to the needs of those in ethnic communities. Racial tension focuses attention not only on the different beliefs and value systems of others but also on how those in ethnic groups view Western approaches to a wide range of things such as, work, leisure, health and illness.

Race, however, is often used interchangeably (and incorrectly) with ethnicity, although race is a scientifically discredited term often used to describe biologically distinct groups of people alleged to have characteristics of an unalterable nature (Montagu, 1997). Banton (1965) provides a clear account of the problematic nature of race, pointing out that to a great extent 'race' is a socially constructed term used to describe specific characteristics of particular groups.

Evidence from the racist murder of Stephen Lawrence, the black student, in South London in 1993 and the subsequent report placed the blame for not solving this crime on the incompetence of the Metropolitan Police and 'institutionalised racism' (Macpherson, 1999). The trial highlighted the racial tension, corruption and prejudice in the Metropolitan Police force. More recently, the treatment of asylum seekers reflects the problematic nature of British attitudes towards those from other cultures and highlights the embedded nature of prejudice and feelings towards those who seek to live in another country. These issues and many others pose enormous political challenges but also cause health care professionals to consider the problem of how to care for and treat those who may be treated with hostility by others in society.

The Problem of Multiculturalism in Britain

Many texts describing health experiences refer to Britain as a multicultural society without addressing some of the fundamental issues of what that really means. The basic assumption being made is that people from different backgrounds, religions, cultures, beliefs and life-styles reside in Britain. But what does it mean in terms of life and health experiences and, more importantly perhaps, how can public health meet the needs of so many different groups?

Multiculturalism refers to the policy of accommodating and assimilating any number of distinct cultures within one society without discrimination. In contemporary Britain this assumption is largely problematic mainly because of rising tensions in intercultural living. The sense of identity we share as host nation and the shared understandings we have of the world, provide meaning and reason to our existence since we invariably encounter others who share the same ideas, customs, values and beliefs about the world. On the one hand Britain as an island is shared by people from many cultures and whether the various groups have shared understandings is a different matter. Perhaps, as Gerrish *et al.* (1996) point out, more accurately, it may be useful to use the term 'multiethnic' to describe the experiences of people in Britain today. Moreover, in a truly multicultural society we should be able to meet others from different cultures and acknowledge, celebrate and share their 'world view' or sense of identity. This popular notion of multiculturalism in Britain, suggesting we share diversity and adopt policies of assimilation leading to antiracism, is not borne out by the evidence. In many parts of Britain there are indications that people know little about other cultures and show little desire to learn (Culley, 1996).

The Government's view suggests that people from ethnic minorities should integrate into the mainstream culture. Government thinking encourages ethnic minority group members to 'accommodate themselves' into British culture in order that they adapt and change, as with people from all cultures, the ideology being to inculcate a sense of Britishness. It has even been suggested that we adopt the American view and introduce naturalisation examinations to allow others to demonstrate their allegiance to the dominant British culture.

The Home Secretary David Blunkett, in a statement in Belgium made the assertion that Asians in the UK should confine themselves to marrying partners in Britain and compared Muslim arranged marriages with practices in medieval England: 'I don't preach that people should have to accept our culture, but that they understand how best to accommodate theirs to living in this country, accepting those broader values which make it possible for us to live together' (*Guardian*, 1 June 2002). Currently the situation with asylum seekers highlights tensions about the right approach to take concerning people from other European countries. This tension reflects negative attitudes and a reluctance to develop intercultural contact with those from other cultures. The riots in Oldham and Brixton are evidence of the difficulties of living in harmony as an integrated society.

Globalisation

The term globalisation was first coined by two Japanese management experts in the early 1980s in an article in the *Harvard Business Review*. Since then it has become common currency in both academic circles and popular parlance. Globalisation has been promoted as a new vision; very similar to the enlightenment period in Europe in the eighteenth century. Globalisation brings the hope of progress and new benefits. As Lee (2000) points out: 'Globalisation is a term which has been used frequently in recent times to describe a wide range of processes and events in the health field. As a convenient catch all. It has been cited as both cause and effect of many things' (p. 6).

During the late 1980s and early 1990s, a series of events including the break up of the Soviet Union, the expansion of the Pacific rim economies and the development of European integration transformed the international environment for trade and investment. This was coupled with a massive increase in technology and the expansion of innovations such as the world wide web (www) and the internet. Barriers of trade, time differences and culture no longer isolated national and international business markets. In many cases nation states were weakened by internal conflict such as civil wars and unrest among the population. These huge changes were influential in the development of a world economic growth particularly in Europe, North America and Japan. As Lee (2000) points out, globalisation is not just about economies and power in different countries but is a process of closer interaction of human activity, with spatial dimensions (concerned with changes to how we experience and perceive human space), temporal dimensions (concerned with changes to the actual and perceived time in which interaction takes places) and cognitive dimensions (changes to the creation and exchange of knowledge, ideas norms beliefs and cultural identities).

Global Public Health

Disease patterns across the world are influenced by increased global mobility. The spread of cholera, TB and the various global flu epidemics that 'jump continents' is a good example (Lee and Dodgson, 1998).

The spread of communicable diseases such as cholera and tuberculosis has resulted from increased geographical mobility as well as recurrent exposure to a broad spectrum of antibiotic drugs. TB is one of the most neglected areas of public health and a major worldwide problem which is out of control in many countries. The WHO declared a TB epidemic in April 1993 and produced a handbook on global TB control (WHO, 1998) to promote effective control of the disease, many of the key principles of which are illustrated in Table 4.2.

Tuberculosis among adults is the leading cause of death in the world due to a single infective agent. In the developing world it causes more than 25 per cent of avoidable adult deaths. Its notification in London (UK) continues to rise (Hayward, 1998) and the global incidence of TB in 1995 was estimated at 8.8 million cases (154 per 1000). Projections in 1994 suggest that TB incidence might increase to 11.9 million cases by 2005. TB rates in London have increased considerably over the last ten years (rates having doubled in many boroughs). The reasons why TB has risen in London are illustrated in Table 4.3.

A few people come to the UK seeking treatment. These numbers do not contribute statistically to the increased numbers seen. The focus on TB is important since it exemplifies how disease such as this can have a major impact on the mental health of people from outside and inside the UK.

Table 4.2   Principles and practical approaches to TB control

Who	Individual rights	Responsibilities
Individuals	Facilitated access to understandable services including information education Effective diagnosis and treatment Effective and safe protection from infection and reinfection (BCG and prophylaxis)	Complete treatment Community benefit from appropriate take up of of BCG immunisation
Families and other community contacts	Screening and other prophylaxis Appropriate treatment	Co-operation and adherence
New arrivals Socially excluded populations, for example, homeless and HIV, prisoners and refugees	Equal rights for best treatment Appropriate and sensitive screening	Early presentation with symptoms Protection of others Completion of treatment
Hospitals and trusts in the UK	Equitable funding mechanisms that reflect local prevalence and populations at risk	Deliver cost-effective treatment programmes Well managed clinical networks Active audit Trained health workers Effective implementation of workplace health and safety policies Occupational health and infection control advice

Source: WHO (1998).

Table 4.3   Reasons for the projected increase in TB in London

---

- Infection recently acquired abroad becomes clinically manifest after arrival in UK
- Latent infection, acquired abroad either recently or in the distant past is reactivated due to the stress/circumstances of immigration
- People arriving in the UK arrive healthy but become infected/reinfected in the UK because of poor housing, overcrowding or poor work conditions

---

Source: Parson, L. and Atkinson, S. (2000) Global and local governance for Tuberculosis. In Parsons, L. and Lister, G. (eds) *Global health: a local issue*. The Nuffield Trust/Royal College of Physicians. London: 134–40.

Many factors play a part in its spread that are closely related to the experiences of ethnic minority groups. However, when we examine the way in which traditional ethnic groups exist outside the mainstream culture we see evidence of a reversal of the trend caused by globalisation whereby people experience the limits of Western medicine and adopt a more traditional approach.

Chinese Culture: the Manchester Model

The Chinese community in Manchester is both diverse and important since little is known about the richness of this particular group who have made up an increasing number of the population since the Second World War. Traditional Chinese groups exist throughout Britain but are more apparent in Manchester where they continue to live outside the confines of a traditional Western way of life and, interestingly, outside the restraint of medical ideology.

Of all the recent ethnic groups of this country, the Chinese are least known. This is partly due to the fact that they are few in number. It is estimated (at the lower level) that there are 3 million people of ethnic minority origin residing in England and Wales – 6 per cent of the total population – but that the Chinese constitute only 0.3 per cent. They are also 0.3 per cent of Greater Manchester, but 0.8 per cent in Manchester itself. Manchester, after London, has the second largest congregation of Chinese, mostly from Hong Kong, but the Manchester population is the fastest growing. The Chinese rarely enter into the politics of the public arena of race relations. They prefer the policy of 'bending with the wind' and not drawing attention to themselves. According to the 1991 census, the Chinese had, percentage wise, two and a half times more than all the other ethnic groups in the socio-economic status I: professional and managerial occupations, and also fewest in category V: unskilled and unemployed. Over 60 per cent could be classified as white-collar workers.

Table 4.4   Chinese population in Britain

Years	China	Hong Kong	Malaysia	Singapore
1951	8 636	3 459	4 046	3 255
1961	9 192	10 222	9 516	9 820
1971	13 495	29 520	25 680	27 335
1981	17 569	58 917	45 430	32 447
1991	18 507	53 473	15 153	4 858

Source: Census Reports for England and Wales 1951–91.

Migration has long been a significant feature of Chinese history. During the political turmoil of pre-Communism, those in North China (Mandarin speaking) migrated to the South to avoid disasters of flooding, earthquakes, drought and the chaos of warlords. As Table 4.4 illustrates, they have had a long migration history with Southeast Asia.

The early Chinese immigrants in the UK were mostly seamen; official reference to their coming as employees of the British East India Company, can be traced to 1814.

Manchester immigrants have a well-defined cultural identity (so have those resident elsewhere). The majority are from Hong Kong, although some were born in Communist China; 90 per cent are Cantonese speaking, only 6 per cent Mandarin speaking (the language of North China and also the official national language) and some Hakka (dialect). Although the majority of respondents reported no religious faith, this is misleading. Most practice versions of Buddhism and Taoism (similar to the way the Japanese mix Buddhism, Christianity and Shintoism – their birth ceremony is Buddhist and funeral rites are Shinto). The common gods the Chinese worship are Wong Tai Sin and Kwan Yum, whose statue or picture is placed in a sacred part of the home; their installation necessitates a special ritual. It is not uncommon to find two or more religions co-existing within the same family. Filial piety is very strong; parents are venerated not only when alive, but also when dead.

Kinship and Family Networks

In Manchester the full range of kinship terminology and its accompanying etiquette is recognised, despite the absence of the complete kinship network. Each family has its own title. A junior member must never shout out the name of a senior member without his or her title. When greeting an elder whom you do not know, the title Shuk/Pak (uncle) is used. A clan refers to those who once lived in the same village in Hong Kong, sharing the same 'surname' of their common ancestor. For example, in Tai Po Lam village (New Territories) most share the same name – Lam – and those of the same generation refer to themselves as 'Tong' (brothers/sisters), using a classificatory kinship terminology. An unknown Chinese without your clan name is referred to as 'Beil' (cousin). Like many members of ethnic groups such as Muslims and Hindus, the Chinese rarely discuss their own family matters with 'non-related' Chinese, let alone strangers like health professionals. The presence of interpreters, especially if known within the Chinese community, will rarely lift the veil of 'family secrecy'. To persist strongly in trying to extract the facts of an illness, as a stranger, is regarded as bad manners and with hostility. Similarly, strangers must not pay a parent the 'compliment' of saying 'what a beautiful/healthy child you have'. This is regarded as an invitation for 'malevolent forces' to target the child. To refer to a child as unpleasant/ugly will 'fool' such external agencies.

Traditional Chinese Medicine

Traditional China was a literate society; hence the coherence of its medical thought is easily traceable through well-prepared documents. The Yellow Emperor (Huang Di) instituted himself as the supreme ruler. The first Chinese medical text – 'The Yellow Emperor's Internal Classic' (Huang Di Nei Jing, *c.* 2852 BC), afterwards referred to as Nei Jing – contains the core of today's medical reasoning.

As Wen-Shing Tseng (1973:569) reminds us: '… in contrast to Western medicine, Chinese medicine evolved in relative isolation with little outside interference and has maintained its coherence throughout its development'. This is not to exert a claim for uniqueness. Traditional Chinese medicine's (TCM's) application of opposites, 'hot' and 'cold' as a universal taxonomic ordering (not only climate, but self, food, season and illness orientation, and so on), is found in other health belief models, as in Latin America (pre-conquest). Ayervedic medicine, India's ancient version, relies for explanatory hue, like TCM, on universal elements of metal, wood, fire, water and earth; both also appeal to astrological influences.

The principles of TCM are widely diffused. Folklore is resplendent with stories of illness and the therapeutic use of medicinal plants. The 'Classic Book of Herbal Medicine' (first century AD) noted that angelica (especially from the Gansu region) had long been used to cure period pains. The distinction between food and medicine could be nonexistent. Pillsbury (1978) described how women 'did the month' after childbirth, keeping free of cold air and drinking ginger-vinegar tea to restore body harmony. Chinese medicine is based on observations of changes in nature. As McNamera and Song Xuan Ke (1995) note:

> nos in miniature. The universe is an
> the Universe. Just as the earth contains
> fluids and blood. And just as the earth
> :cted by internal weathers. (p. 27)

ing, its Qi is warm; fire represents
ng summer, its Qi is damp; metal
r represents winter, its Qi is cold.
he gall bladder as judge; lung as
soul; and liver a military com-
ess. Each of nature's spirits com-
ith the heart; wind with the liver;
ourg's interviewees born in Hong
taying one's life' – moderation in
mper and maintain family har-
M, as part of nature, are widely
is the hearth is the material and
oups were a dominant means of
itions produced by some agency
ood condition are notable exam-
major axes of bodily functions.
1 to share the happiness of a new
gui is a common blood tonic for
inese also believe that the longer
ve. That the soup's vitamins will
t within the concepts of TCM.
e Chinese population living in
one survey, found that 32.5 per
wo-week period. Chinese med-
than Western preparations with
e of information about drugs.
f self medication is often based
o for his/her health and illness,
ffective and they have a good
ı some of the commercial prod-
ors expressed concern that there
cts. Thus it would be wise for
t's history to explore the use of
n be heavily laced with caffeine
ın Taiwan.

Mental Health

Mental illness among Chinese people is considered more stigmatising than in the West and the Government has been reluctant to have open debate on this issue. The 'shame' of mental illness is not only a family matter but is also considered to reflect badly on the Government. As Pearson (1995) points out, foreign visitors to China must still make a health declaration with psychosis bracketed with AIDS and leprosy as diseases to be questioned. Overseas researchers into mental illness are strongly restricted, unlike those into general medicine, for example 'high-tech' medicine. Traditional Chinese medicine has no significant recognition of mental illness. Chinese knowledge never underwent a Cartesian revolution, introducing a body/mind split. TCM is completely holistic. Dian kuang is recognised only as an 'extreme' behavioural condition, totally inappropriate for the continuity of everyday interaction, often based on 'rules of etiquette'. Chinese pharmaceutics also never developed remedies for the range of mental illnesses found in the West. The *Nei Jing*, for many years China's most popular medical text, refers to the condition of dian kuang, known colloquially as 'crazy'. Imposing Western *etic* categories, it is possible to recognise kuang as 'psychosis' – people believing themselves to be famous lords, being able to perform ecstatic acts of flying over mountains, and so on. The dian component is comparable with a deep depression, from which there is no recovery.

As the previous account has shown, definitions and experiences of health and illness are very much influenced by cultural orientation. The account of the Chinese community in Manchester illustrates that, like many ethnic groups, religion and morality form 'rules of living' and are prominent in their health belief systems. Despite their proximity to and affiliations with Western life, many ethnic groups retain their sense of traditionalism when it comes to health and illness. This may be due to a cultural orientation towards what they experience during their lives as well as their beliefs and attitudes. It is the latter we now turn to as a way of developing greater sensitivity to the health needs of ethnic minority groups in Britain.

The Need for Cultural Sensitivity

As this chapter has shown, the way forward in terms of limiting the inequalities of opportunity for ethnic minority groups in Britain is to understand how and why some people with different cultural perceptions experience poor health. Nurses in particular, as the largest NHS employee, need to become culturally competent; that is, to become aware of their own cultural background and values and to develop knowledge of information specific to other cultures. The ability of health practitioners to interact successfully with those from ethnic minorities depends on the professional's awareness of the lay beliefs, values and attitudes of those who have wide and varied perceptions of health and illness (Henley, 1979). In particular, health care professionals who are not immune to stereotyping patients should avoid blaming patients for their own illness because of the patients' life-styles, for example, the Afro-Caribbean Rastafarian who develops lung cancer as a result of excessively smoking 'ganja'.

One of the key ways in which public health for those at the cultural margins of society can improve and become sustained is through a greater push towards cultural awareness and sensitivity. This we argue can take place by tackling three major issues. First, to challenge racism, on an individual level and perhaps more importantly the institutionalised racism that forms part of the fabric of public services. Second, to de-emphasise 'victim blaming' and shift the focus on the underlying social and economic issues which prevail in society and cause many people from other cultures to live second-class lives. Finally, to highlight and acknowledge cultural diversity. This can be achieved in a number of ways, largely through education with schools taking a major role and, in particular, health and public service providers encouraging and appreciating differences in social life and their role in helping others to develop a sense of their own cultural identity without the need to feel that they have to make choices about where their affiliations lie. Understanding the beliefs of other cultures is a step towards developing greater awareness and nurses embracing a holistic approach to health care. Table 4.5 provides a broad overview of the health beliefs of others, contrasting internal belief systems with externalising approaches. The Chinese operate within a health belief, referred to as 'externalising'. The causation of illness is primarily located outside the body; illness can be precipitated by the seasons, climate or astrological positions of the stars. This contrasts with Western biomedical approaches based on an internalising health belief model, where illness causation rests largely within the body. However, both models accept that to be healthy is the ideal: healthy also implies to be in harmony. Knowledge about health and illness in cultures with external belief systems see numerous ways of healing from lay preachers to witchdoctors and self-healing, rather than the narrowly focused view of Western medicine with the power in the hands of the specialists.

The need for cultural sensitivity in relation to people from diverse communities has never been more important, particularly in light of recent events in Britain surrounding the continuing problems of asylum seekers. The latter throws into relief a range of problems relating to attitudes towards members of other cultures. In relation to the fiasco that resulted from the Stephen Lawrence murder, Stowell-Smith and McKeown (2001)

Public Health and Society

Table 4.5   Internalised and externalised health beliefs

	Internalising	*Externalising*
Source of illness	Within the body, for example, a virus	Outside the body, for example, tension in relationships breaking moral codes
Causation	Multiple	Fewer, for example, the same cause having multiple disease effects
Proof of improvement	Empirical science	Symbolic
Body	Complex physical	Simple, for example, the body differentiation is often a 'black box' and a receptacle for disease
Practitioner	Treats the individual client: passivity	Treats the individual as part of sets of expected relationships to reconcile disharmony
Health knowledge	Monopoly of specialists	Widely dispersed in society giving clients great influence as healers
Society	Complex division of labour producing economic surpluses that support the elite	Simple division of labour, very little surplus, very small 'leisured' elite or 'literati'
Recovery from illness	When fit for work	When restored to the moral order of the group, for example, the Cheyenne have a 7-day singing ceremony for the ill, each verse historically recreating the universe; then the sick person is finally incorporated into it

Source: Adapted from Young, A. (1976) Internalising and externalising medical belief systems: an Ethiopian example. *Social Science and Medicine*, 10, 147–56.

point out that the issue of institutionalised racism highlights the need for greater cultural competence while drawing our attention to what they refer to as 'racialised government rhetoric' about the way we need to treat asylum seekers. The issue of asylum seekers is a revealing example of ethnocentricity and reveals how, as a society, we fail to put into practice what politicians and others consistently point out to be politically correct. It also highlights how, when faced with 'hard issues', racial differences and prejudice come out as very worrying and powerful forces in our dealing with others for whom we appear to have no clear affinity.

Conclusion

This chapter has argued that ethnic minority groups in Britain experience inequalities in health and are vulnerable in terms of their lack of ability to access and effectively use health resources. This may not be due to deficiencies in their ability to assimilate the dominant culture, due to the dominance of a Westernised medical approach focusing on internal models of illness causation. Moreover, the evidence suggests that it is our lack of understanding of their beliefs which constrain them from adapting to a new culture. The many global changes taking place throughout the world help to create the illusion that the world is getting smaller, but attitudes, beliefs and values for many people from ethnic minorities have their origins in traditional approaches, as the description of Chinese people in Manchester depicted. The more sinister problems associated with prejudice need to be tackled at all levels bearing in mind that many problems are encountered within our institutions. In order to remain sensitive to the health needs of others, work at a global political, economic and social level needs to take place. At the same time there is a need to conduct further research and to ensure that the results are made available and are implemented on a large scale. The authors call for all readers to become culturally competent and adopt sensitive cultural standards, that is, the standards we use to assess ourselves and others. These consist of widely held beliefs about what we consider worthwhile, desirable or important for well-being. What is important about addressing the health needs of diverse ethnic groups is that health care practitioners should strive to avoid the narrow ethnocentric view encapsulated in Western bio-medical approaches and in doing so become sensitive and responsive to the diversity and richness of different cultures.

References

Acheson, D. (1988) *Independent enquiry into inequalities in health.* London: Stationery Office.
Amin, K. and Oppenheim, C. (1992) *Poverty in black and white: deprivation and ethnic minorities.* London: CPAG.
Banton, M.P. (1965) *Roles: an introduction to the study of social relations.* London: Tavistock.
Beaglehole, R. and Bonita, R. (1997) *Public health at the crossroads.* Cambridge, UK: Cambridge University Press.
Bott, E. (1971) *Family and social network.* London: Tavistock.
Bourne, J. (1994) Facts and figures. In Bourne, J., Bridges, L. and Searle, C. (eds) *Outcast England: how schools exclude black children.* London: Institute of Race Relations.
Bourne, J., Bridges, L. and Searle, C. (1994) *Outcast England: how schools exclude black children.* London: Institute of Race Relations.
Culley, L. (1996) A critique of multiculturalism in health care: the challenge for nurse education. *Journal of Advanced Nursing,* 23, 564–70.
Field, D. and Taylor, S. (1995) (eds) *Sociology of health and health care.* London: Blackwell.

Furnham, A. and Bochner, S. (1990) *Culture shock: psychological reactions to unfamiliar environments.* London: Routledge.

Gerrish, K. (2000) Researching ethnic diversity in the British NHS: methodological and practical concerns. *Journal of Advanced Nursing*, 31, 918–25.

Gerrish, K., Husband, C. and Mackenzie, J. (1996) *Nursing for a multi-ethnic society.* Buckingham: Open University Press.

Gluckman, M. (1964) *Closed systems and Open Minds: the Limits of Naivety in Social Anthropology.* Edinburgh: Oliver and Boyd.

Hayward, A. (1998) Tuberculosis control in London – the need for change. A report for the Thames Regional Directors of Public Health. Discussion document. NHS Executive.

Henley, A. (1979) *Asian patients in hospital and home.* London: Pitman Medical Library.

Howitt, D. and Owusu-Bempah, K. (1999) Education psychology and the construction of black childhood. *Education and child psychology*, 16, 3, 17–29.

Jary, D. and Jary, J. (2000) *Sociology* (3rd edn), Glasgow: Harper Collins.

Lam, C.L.K., Catarivas, M.G., Munro, C. and Lauder, I.J. (1994) Self-medication among Hong Kong Chinese. *Social Science and Medicine*, 9, 1641–47.

Lee, K. (2000) The global dimensions of health. In Parsons, L. and Lister, G (eds) *Global health: a local dimension.* London: The Nuffield Trust, 6–18.

Lee, K. and Dodgson, R. (1998) Globalisation and Cholera: implications for global governance. Paper presented to the British International Studies Association annual conference, University of Sussex, Falmer, December 1998.

Lister, G. (2000) Rising awareness of public health. In Parsons, L. and Lister, G. (eds) *Global health: a local issue.* London: The Nuffield Trust/Royal College of Physicians.

Lister, G. (2001) Global health: implications for policy. In Parsons, L. and Lister, G. (eds) *Global health: a local issue.* London: The Nuffield Trust/Royal College of Physicians, 19–33.

Macpherson, W. (1999) *The Stephen Lawrence inquiry: report of an inquiry.* London: Home Office.

Mahoney, T. (1988) *Governing schools: powers, issues and practice.* London: Macmillan, now Palgrave.

McNamera, S. and Song Xuan, Ke (1995) *Traditional Chinese Medicine.* London: Hamish Hamilton.

Montagu, A. (1997) *Man's most dangerous myth: the fallacy of race.* 6th edn, Walnut Creek: Alta Maria Press.

Nehru, J. (1936) *An autobiography.* London: Bodley Head (reprinted, 1958).

Owusu-Bempah, K. and Howitt, D. (2000) *Psychology beyond Western Perspectives.* London: BPS.

Parson, L. and Atkinson, S. (2000) Global and local governance for Tuberculosis. In Parsons, L. and Lister, G. (eds) *Global health: a local issue.* London: The Nuffield Trust/Royal College of Physicians, 134–40.

Pearson, V. (1995) *Mental Health Care in China. State Policies, Professional Services and Family Responsibilities.* London: Gaskell.

Peterson, A. and Lupton, D. (1996) *The new Public Health.* London: Sage.

Pillsbury, B. (1978) 'Doing the month': Confinement and convalescence of Chinese women after childbirth. *Social Science and Medicine*, 12, 11–22.

Radcliff-Brown, A. (1956) *African systems of kinship and marriage.* Oxford: Oxford University Press.

Richman, J. (1987) *Medicine and health.* London: Longman.

Seebohn Report (1968) *Re-organisation of social services.* London: Department of Health.

Stowell-Smith, M. and McKeown, M. (2001) Race, stigma and stereotyping. In Mason, T. Carlisle, C., Watkins C. and Whitehead, E. (eds) *Stigma and Social Exclusion.* London: Routledge, 158–69.

Ward, L. (1967) Some observations of the underlying dynamics of conflict in a foreign student. *Journal of the American College Health Association*, 10, 430–40.

Wen-Shin Tseng (1973) The development of psychiatric concepts in traditional Chinese medicine. *Archives of General Psychiatry*, 29, 569–75.

WHO (1983) *Depression and disorder in different cultures.* Geneva: World Health Organisation.

WHO (1998) *Tuberculosis handbook.* Geneva: WHO.

Wilmot, P. and Young, M. (1960) *Family and class in a London suburb.* London: Routledge and Kegan Paul.

Zwingmann, C.A.A. and Gunn, A.D.G. (1983) *Uprooting and health; psychological problems of students from abroad.* Geneva: World Health Organisation, Division of Mental Health.

5

Access to Health Care: Vulnerable Groups in Society

MARYAM SPANSWICK

The key points discussed in this chapter include:

- external and internal concepts of vulnerability from different perspectives
- the significant factors that influence the degree of vulnerability experienced by different groups
- the serious implications that vulnerability has for the person, their family and society.

Introduction

Understanding the concept of vulnerability is important because of its implications and the way it permeates and influences every aspect of life, including people's health and social welfare. The experience of vulnerability causes stress and anxiety, which affects the person's psychological, physical and social well-being. Although everyone is vulnerable at different times in their life, the circumstances of some people's lives mean they are more vulnerable than others and more likely to move along a downward spiral in a society that cannot cope with 'difference'. This chapter will concentrate on the aspects that make individuals and groups vulnerable. The chapter will also explore briefly which groups may be considered vulnerable and why, and finally the chapter will consider some of the common denominators of vulnerability which may assist in developing a strategy of prevention and protection.

Briggs (1961) identifies three principal elements of the welfare state:

1 a guarantee of minimum standards, including a minimum income

2 social protection in the event of insecurity

3 the provision of services at the best level possible.

This has become identified in practice with the institutional model of welfare. The key elements are social protection and the provision of welfare services on the basis of right. However, in a system that was created to provide a framework of equality and equity, the post-modern welfare state has arguably been unable to keep abreast of its goals. It is clearly debatable whether social protection and provision of welfare services are available as a 'right' and indeed perspective and position in society are likely to influence people's opinions of whether they should be.

The NHS in particular finds itself in the difficult situation of trying to obviate, for example, the 'postcode lottery', as it is called in the media, and yet at the same time tailor health solutions to particular areas according to needs assessments. It is also trying to provide care and treatment according to patient and client views and simultaneously to use only evidence-based practice approved by the National Institute of Clinical Excellence (NICE). Financial limitations do not always allow for the provision of services that are deemed 'non-essential'. For example, there is no national policy of agreement regarding funding of fertility treatments, which results in differences in service availability and charges to the general public. Despite the attempt to encourage local public involvement in determining local needs, the process is not always flexible and open to debate. In general the reasons for inequity in services are complex and not always obvious. However, they are further compounded by the fact that there are individuals within society who experience increased difficulties in gaining access to public services, including the most basic form of health care, because of their personal circumstances. Within the literature reviewed, such individuals are often referred to as 'vulnerable populations'.

Vulnerability – its Definition and Characteristics

A review of the literature reveals how frequently the term 'vulnerability' appears in nursing terminology and literature. However, the concept is neither clear nor comprehensive in its definition and there appears to be a limited consensus of opinion with regard to a precise definition. Although it is a vague concept and open to a variety of definitions and interpretations, implicit in the idea is the notion of danger or risk, whether it is a reality based one or something the person fears. With this in mind, it may be argued that, as individuals, we are all vulnerable, but clearly some members of society are more vulnerable than others. The notion of vulnerability has been linked with a susceptibility to or risk of ill health and/or stress (Philips, 1992). The term has also been used to describe how an individual's personal characteristics and their relationship to environmental factors may influence health (Rose and Killien, 1983). Other definitions associate vulnerability with issues of defencelessness and weakness and an inability to protect personal welfare and rights. Rogers (1997) states that the use of the term vulnerability implies that an individual, family unit or social group is susceptible to health problems, injury, danger, loss or neglect. The definition and understanding of vulnerability may be substantiated further or given more meaning if it is conceptualised as a continuum that is dynamic and constantly changing, with individuals at different points on the continuum at different times (Rose and Killien, 1983; Copp, 1986; Rogers, 1997). An individual's point on any continuum is influenced by a series of complex interactions between internal and external factors rather than a straightforward sum of these factors (Appleton, 1994). Examples of internal factors include self-esteem, social support networks, personal relationships and degree of health and well-being. External factors might include issues such as housing, financial circumstances, employment status and certainly level of control over life circumstances.

Within the literature, vulnerability is often described in terms of, or used interchangeably with, the concept of risk. As with the concept of vulnerability, the notion of risk is open to some ambiguous interpretation. There is an abundance of references around the concept of risk within the fields of mental health nursing and child protection, but the meaning is implied rather than clarified. Rose and Killien (1983) have differentiated between the concepts of risk and vulnerability, describing risk as the presence of potentially stressful factors in a person's environment which are dangerous to health, and vulnerability as personal factors that interact with the environment to influence health. They also suggest that 'at risk' is used to determine the likelihood of an event occurring or to distinguish people who may develop problems in the future. Rose and Killien go on to suggest that risk and vulnerability are interconnected with one affecting the other in a dynamic way in that the characteristics of both person and environment influence health and illness. Rogers (1997) and Philips (1992) both support the tangible relationship between risk and vulnerability and stress the importance of considering both personal and environmental factors when assessing clients' health needs. The ambiguity of the term vulnerability and the fact that it may be interpreted in different ways within the nursing community illustrates one of the fundamental problems in trying to apply such an abstract concept to nursing practice.

Spiers (2000) identifies the possibility of an 'emic' perspective (where vulnerability is based on the experience of challenges to one's integrity) and an 'etic' perspective (based on demographic characteristics which assign a person to a particular group with a higher probability of health or social problems). Spiers suggests that the etic perspective should be rebadged as 'at risk' as it serves to identify groups of people for whom services can be judged at a reasonably collective level. However, the emic perspective is a dimension of quality of life which is about the experience that an individual goes through as they recognise the challenges to their hoped for quality of life. When assessing community health needs it is this emic perspective which may be lost in the anxiety to identify those 'at risk'. This goes some way to explaining why some people when faced with similar circumstances become more vulnerable than others. However, Spiers' notion of emic perspective also lends itself to viewing those who fall victim to vulnerability as being unable to cope, weak, and perhaps easier to place into the category of dependent and in need of professional support and help and all that goes with it.

From a health perspective we arguably have a view of vulnerability as transient, that is, individuals or groups in circumstances which are currently placing them at risk but for which there are interventions which may work towards alleviating the problems. This notion is what could be argued to underpin the public health approach to vulnerability. There is however a rather more hard edged sociological perspective which may recognise the vulnerability as vulnerability to devaluation (and indeed social exclusion as identified in the chapter by Costello).

Wolfensberger (1987) does not take such a sympathetic view of the way that society treats vulnerable people. He offers a chilling context for vulnerability to be constructed in Western society. First, he identifies how there is inevitably a lust for power in human societies which invariably results in some form of stratification. He gives a vision of how a society may work more towards creating rather than relieving vulnerability thus:

> Stratification means that a society is horizontally divided: some people rise to the top, some remain in the middle and some end up on the bottom. Almost invariably, only a few will be on the top; the rest of society may bulge at the bottom, as most societies have done, or in the middle as ours does. This stratification is attained and maintained by peoples' pursuit and use of power. Power consists of the ability to control others. To a very large extent, this power is based on control over people's livelihood, their economic resources, their bodily security, their abode, their esteem in the eyes of others and their relationships. People are largely controlled by their fears that they might lose whichever of these they cherish, and most people cherish all of them. All this means that in a stratified system, those on the top possess and wield the greatest amount of power (Wolfensberger 1987:4).

Wolfensberger identifies how societies place devalued people into categories such as 'sub-human', 'animal', 'menace', 'evil' and other equally devalued labels. When an individual is consigned to such a category it gives society 'permission' to treat them badly. Wolfensberger's work is interesting when we look at the behaviour of the media in Britain today and the language used to describe certain vulnerable groups which then creates a culture of 'permission' to think the unthinkable. As an example we need only look at the language used in the early days of HIV disease and, today, the language used about asylum seekers and even those living on welfare benefit. Wolfensberger identifies the potential groups of de-valued people (see Table 5.1).

The single biggest predictor of who will be devalued in a society is the prevailing value system of that society. A society that values physical beauty, for example, will devalue those who are 'ugly'. A society that values wealth will devalue the poor and so on. With some reflection on Wolfensberger's work we may begin to recognise 'vulnerable' as synonymous with 'devalued'. What becomes clearer is that as they become more

Table 5.1 Minority groups widely devalued in Western societies

Those handicapped in:
- sense: vision, hearing
- body: cerebral palsy, epilepsy, paralysis, amputation
- mind: retarded, disordered (*sic*)

Those disordered in conduct/behaviour:
- activity level: hyperactive, lethargic
- sexual orientation or conduct
- self-destructive, 'substance' dependent

The socially rebellious:
- dissident
- work resistive
- lawless, delinquent, imprisoned

The poor

Those with few or unwanted skills:
- illiterate
- unemployed

Those unassimilated for other reasons:
- age: unborn, aged
- race: nationality, ethnicity
- religion

Source: Wolfensberger (1987).

and more alienated by a society (which is the danger identified by Wolfensberger), vulnerable people will find themselves in a situation in which improvement becomes an uphill struggle against increasing odds. One situation will impact on another, which then worsens and impacts on further aspects of the vulnerable person's life. To explore how this happens to people and some of the difficulties that ensue, a case study will be used which will highlight some of the issues driving people further and further into vulnerability.

Jane

Jane is a 28-year-old single mother with three children aged 9 years, 6 years and 6 months. She left school at 16 with no qualifications and went to work in a retail outlet. She gave up this work when she became pregnant at 18 years old and has not had a job since, as she has no one to care for the children while she goes out to work. The father of Jane's baby did not want to offer any support and her two other children are the result of previous relationships. Jane's housing benefit has gradually been reduced over time. Her private landlord decided to stop renting the property when the lease came up for renewal and with reduced housing benefit Jane could no longer afford either the private rent or the deposit that would be required on a new rental.

Jane has been offered council accommodation but the offers were for areas that have problems with anti-social behaviour and are miles away from her only support who is her mother. She is now not being offered any further properties because of her refusals and has had arguments with the housing officer who finds Jane a 'nuisance' and is unwilling to help her any further. Jane has also been offered the homeless families unit but this has problems with drug use and Jane is unwilling to take her children there as she feels this will put them in danger and put them under a 'bad influence'. As a result she is living in a caravan in her mother's garden and the children are living with her mother and two sisters in the house which is now overcrowded with no room for Jane. Jane feels that she is losing control over the care of her children, she is drinking in the evenings and has now been diagnosed with post-natal depression.

There are several issues which merit some further exploration as factors which drive people further and further into vulnerability. First, the notion of poverty and economic inequality within a society of plenty. Second, the powerlessness and lack of control that is clearly felt by Jane and how this spirals the vulnerable individual downwards into incrementally worsening situations. Finally, the issue of social support: whether this is at the individual or the community level and how crucial this can be in reducing the impact of the vulnerability on an individual or group.

Poverty and Economic Inequality

Jane may or may not be described as poor depending upon who makes the assessment. Poverty and its measurement have a long history of semantic problems. The United Kingdom has no officially agreed definition of poverty and therefore poverty and its measurement appear to be ad hoc with assessments of poverty arbitrarily concluded to be based on the notion of low comparative income. Piachaud (1981) argues that the definition of poverty is a moral question, that it refers to hardship and that is unacceptable. Poverty may refer to:

- material conditions – needing goods and services, multiple deprivation, or a low standard of living

- economic position – low income, limited resources, inequality or low social class

- social position of the poor through lack of entitlement, dependency or social exclusion.

The United Kingdom and 116 other countries made the commitment to eradicate absolute poverty and significantly reduce overall poverty as defined by the United Nations (UN, 1995), defining absolute poverty as:

A condition characterised by severe deprivation of basic human needs, including food, safe drinking water, sanitation facilities, health, shelter, education and information. It depends not only on income but also on access to services. (UN, 1995:57)

and overall poverty as:

Lack of income and productive resources to ensure sustainable livelihoods; hunger and malnutrition; ill health; limited or lack of access to education and other basic services; increased morbidity and mortality from illness, homelessness and inadequate housing; unsafe environments and social discrimination and exclusion. It is also characterised by lack of participation in decision making and in civil social and cultural life. (UN, 1995:57)

Poverty brings with it a downward spiral of circumstances that serve only to increase vulnerability and it is easy to see from the report by Gordon *et al.* (2000) how this may result in the poor becoming a vulnerable and devalued group. In their report Gordon *et al.* identify that roughly 9.5 million people in Britain today cannot afford adequate housing conditions, 8 million cannot afford one or more essential household goods. Almost 7.5 million people are too poor to engage in common social activities considered necessary by the majority of the population. About two million British children go without at least two things that they need. About 6.5 million adults go without essential clothing and around 4 million are not fed properly by today's standards. It starts to become easy to recognise a connection between this and mental health in terms of depression and how Jane may be diagnosed as post-natally depressed. The risks to this young woman and her children are clear, certainly to their health and safety in the broadest terms.

Poverty and employment go hand in hand. However, poverty is not only the result of unemployment; far from it. The report by Gosling *et al.* (1997) demonstrates that low pay is connected to increased chances of unemployment, to re-employment being at reduced wages and is connected with observable characteristics such as age, gender and educational qualifications. Again, evidence of the vulnerable becoming increasingly vulnerable.

It is widely acknowledged that poverty and ill-health go hand in hand. However, it is a popular misconception that the relationship between ill health and poverty will diminish to the point of extinction as the wealth of a nation improves and cascades down the social scale. The logical conclusion to this problematic relationship is to eradicate poverty and its effects by giving more money to those people who live on or below the economic poverty line and that once everyone achieves certain social standards, ill health will disappear. However, increasing numbers of studies show that fundamental to the experience of good health is income distribution and the most effective approach to reducing health inequalities is through the redistribution of income.

Studies by Wilkinson (1996) highlight that the effects of inequality are more pronounced in societies where there are greater extremes of wealth and poverty than in societies where the spectrum of wealth and poverty is much narrower. For example, within the general population of developing countries the economic differences between those that have and those that do not have is measurably less than in developed countries. In focusing on the degree of intra-nation inequalities rather than the almost irrelevant direct comparison between developing and developed nations and the evidence suggests that developed countries would do well to reduce the differences or inequalities between those that have and those that do not have. Wilkinson goes on to state that by reducing the degree of difference, the effects of inequalities would be less pronounced and also less harmful. The material differences are not in themselves the most important factor in determining health status. For example, the average standard of living in some developed countries is twice as high compared to others, but benefits in improved health status of those wealthier countries are not visible. The important issue here is that the concept of poverty is relative rather than absolute. What creates the damage is less the face-to-face inequality between neighbours, and more the lower status that comes with a person's identity within society at large. It would appear that reduced income inequalities lead to a healthier society, but how can this be explained? The evidence to support the causal relationship between poverty and ill health is difficult to carry out in randomised, scientific experiments, but arguments to support it are there. In less developed countries a clear relationship exists between measures of health such as life expectancy and income. However, the relationship becomes weaker once average income rises beyond a certain point. It becomes more like that of richer industrial and post-industrial countries where health improvements are no longer strongly linked to increasing economic wealth. In fact there is a causal relationship whereby increased unequal wealth distribution leads to increased health differences (Quick and Wilkinson, 1991). Discussions on improving health need to focus less on the amount of money needed to provide minimum material needs and more on what is required to become a valued member of mainstream society where ambition and drive is encouraged and realised.

Wilkinson (1996) suggests that psychological and social health and welfare are most affected by economic inequality, damaging self-confidence, social relations and in turn the very social fabric of society. Retrospective data analysis by Wilkinson (1996) reveals how during the two World Wars mortality and morbidity rates dropped, despite economic hardship, which also saw reduced economic disparity between social classes. Economic inequalities lead to a society of those that have and those that do not have. This in turn cultivates both feelings of resentment from those that do not have towards those that have and feelings of inadequacy in not having. This social divide also perpetuates the circle of poverty down the line of generations of a family.

The nature of the relationship between income inequality and murder appears to be similar to the association there is between mortality and income distribution (Wilkinson, 1996). Societies with a high incidence of murder also have a high incidence of death rates from other causes, which suggests that economic inequalities have a strong bearing on both rates of murder and other causes of death. In trying to understand the relationship, particularly between causes of violence, murder and income inequalities, Gilligan (1996) suggests that the causes of violence and incidence of murder arise from people experiencing strong feelings of shame and humiliation and not feeling respected. No matter how severe the punishment, the act of violence, even to the point of murder, was a means of saving face or self-respect. Sensitivity to the issue of respect and social status is exacerbated by wider differences in income distribution.

Control

Much of what is identified above is evidence of people's lives spiralling out of control. Power is being wielded over vulnerable people which keeps them in a situation of poverty because the powerful groups in society define the criteria for being accepted as a full member of that society and people outside those criteria find that their lives conspire to keep them outside of the accepted group (Wolfensberger, 1987). In Jane's case, she is a single parent (devalued category), she is unemployed (devalued category) and she is homeless (devalued category) and now she has mental health problems (devalued category). Her life is out of control and she does not have the resources to regain that control.

Control or lack of it either in job or home circumstances is recognised to be a determinant in health in studies such as those undertaken by Professor Michael Marmot and colleagues (Bosma *et al.*, 1997). These demonstrated that control over job is an important determinant of coronary heart disease. Control is beginning to be recognised as an important variable in people's health and much of the recent work on stress demonstrates this. In the terms of Antonovsky (1987) (for more detail see Haggart's chapter) people like Jane have their sense of coherence compromised and are therefore unlikely to be able to be healthy (and indeed are much more open to bad things happening to them).

Powerlessness and feelings of powerlessness underpin the theory of locus of control as defined by Rotter (1954) but raised widely in health promotion as a reason for people feeling unable to make any changes in their lives. Powerlessness leads to low self-esteem and certainly will promote anger and occasionally antisocial behaviour. Jane became angry with her housing officer, which led to an argument, accusations and now less likelihood of her achieving her aim of a council home near her mother.

Powerlessness was identified by Seeman and Lewis (1995) as a predictor of psycho-social symptoms, limits to activity, deterioration in health and increased mortality. They identify powerlessness as a significant factor but only part of what happens when people are alienated from society. Wallerstein (1992) also identifies from her review of the research that powerlessness or lack of control over destiny emerges as a broad based risk factor for disease.

There may be some mediating factors to some of the above and one of these is certainly considered to be social support.

Social Support

Consider what may have happened to Jane without the albeit limited social support of her mother. She may have moved to the area with high levels of antisocial behaviour, she would have become lonely and socially isolated, may have made friends with people who behave in a way that she would not have chosen to. All of this would have had an effect on her life expectations as well as the children.

Scientific studies support the theoretical claims that social relationships have a causal impact on health and people's ability to function in society. Early work by Durkheim (1951), suggested that social relationships affected suicide and that socially isolated people were more likely to commit suicide than those more socially integrated individuals (House *et al.*, 1988). There is a significant relationship between an increased mortality rate among persons with a low quantity and, in some cases, quality of relationships. Studies show that not only are more socially integrated people less likely to die, they are also more healthy physically and psychologically (House *et al.*, 1988).

Scientists have long been aware of the relationship between health and social relationships, but the causal relationship has been less clear. Are socially isolated people more likely to become ill and die? Or are unhealthy people less likely to establish and maintain social relationships and contacts? Or is there some other unknown factor, which leads to people having both a lack of social relationships and poor health? Through studies investigating stress and psychosocial factors, it would seem that social support and relationships are protective of health (Cassel, 1976; Cobb, 1976; House, 1981). Within developed countries the incidence of chronic diseases is growing and, to a larger extent, has overtaken the incidence of acute disease. The origins of many disease processes are a result not only of biological factors but also in combination with behavioural and environmental factors over a period of time. While social relationships might serve to promote health, more specifically their main mechanism of protection is thought to be in the way that they diminish or cushion the potentially harmful effects of psychosocial stresses. Studies by Berkman and Syme (1979) assessed individuals for the presence of four family/social ties, which included marriage; extended family/friends contact; church membership and other formal/informal affiliations. The results of this study found that the presence of one or more of these social supports reduced morbidity and mortality rates. The results of this study were supported by the work of House (1981). It is interesting to note that variation was observed by race, sex and geographical location. Male mortality significantly reduced in proportion to the increase in social connections and while women showed a similar relationship, it was weaker and statistically less significant. Despite the overall variation, the trend was consistent in its picture, which showed that social 'connectedness' was a significant predictor of mortality. The mechanisms linking social relationships to health are not clear although it is thought that social relationships have both a physiological and psychological effect.

Animal studies demonstrate that variation in social relationships produce physiological and psychological changes that, if prolonged, could cause serious illness and even death (House *et al.*, 1988). Social relationships encourage the development of a sense of self, which in turn promotes healthy behaviour, choices and approaches to living (Umberson, 1987).

For many vulnerable people, the lack of social support systems that come with having some kind of secure home are their major problem. Unfortunately, growing numbers of our society are being denied the stability of what a home can offer, which is a secure base that is part of community with social relationships. The experience of homelessness is associated with high levels of social exclusion. For example, with no proof of identity or by registering an address as no fixed abode (NFA) can mean individuals being denied access to social and health services that other members of the population take for granted (Grenier, 1996; North *et al.*, 1996). Within the primary health care setting general practitioners (GPs) are the usual point of entry to the health service, but registering with a GP is not always straightforward for a homeless person. So the social support (lack of which is part of the reason the person is vulnerable in the first place) becomes ever more difficult to attain, so ensuring that the person is more likely to be maintained in their vulnerable position.

Evidence demonstrates that between 28 and 37 per cent of the homeless population are not registered with a GP, compared to only 3 per cent of the general population (Big Issue, 1998; Shelter, 1998). The majority of homeless people receive health treatment by accessing secondary care services, that is, accident and emergency (A&E) departments (Black *et al.*, 1991; Victor *et al.*, 1989). Thus vulnerable people make the best use of the resources at their disposal in order to access services that are viewed as a right by the rest of the population. Unfortunately, not only homeless individuals but travellers, refugees and asylum seekers as well as people with mental health problems can be turned away from accident and emergency units. Rather than view this demand as an expressed need (see Horne's chapter on health needs assessment) it is considered 'inappropriate' use.

The Public Health Dimension

So why should society really care about the extent of income inequality and its consequences? Income inequality increases the disparity between social affluence and deprivation and concentrates the effects, which is reflected in the neighbourhoods that develop. Segregated residential areas develop which are largely determined by economic wealth and income and this is a trend that is increasing as disparity of wealth increases (Wacquant and Wilson, 1989). Wealthier areas actively invest in their communities, thereby improving the provision and availability of public services and amenities. While there may be improved or strengthened community relations within these neighbourhoods there is an overall reduced sense of social cohesion within the society at large which affects everybody, no matter how rich or poor they are. Studies by Kaplan *et al.* (1996) reveal that wide income differences co-exist with lack of investment in human capital within poorer areas of society. This in turn leads to increased school drop-out rates, reduced spending on education which affects the quality of the service, reduced literacy rates and increased numbers of poorly educated and unskilled members of society. Again, the fabric of society at large suffers the consequences of this as productivity is reduced which slows overall economic growth. Another consequence of a breakdown in social cohesion through income inequality is the stability of democracy. Putnam's 20-year study of local government performance in Italy (Putnam *et al.*, 1993) revealed that the measure of social cohesion, for example, the strength of citizen participation within society, was a strong predictor of local government performance. Regions of strong social cohesion were more likely to trust fellow citizens, have high levels of mutual tolerance and a high regard for solidarity and equality. Where there were low levels of civic trust, local government performance and voter turnout rates were low. Therefore the election of politicians does not necessarily reflect the democratic will of the population, but rather campaign strategies that are more likely to meet the needs of the socially affluent.

The extent of inequality within society is a consequence of explicit public policies and choice. Therefore it is society's choice about how much inequality it will tolerate, but the results are not isolated to affect only the poorer sections of society – everybody is affected. Reducing inequality and the increasing growth of it improves social cohesion, which in turn improves population health and all this entails.

By acknowledging the relationship between relative deprivation and health, it is simple to understand why low social status and relative poverty carry such great social and health costs. Consequently, it is easy to understand why it is so important to develop appropriate and applicable policies as a means of dealing with the inequalities and the consequences. While reducing income inequality is an important purpose, it would not be beneficial or effective in its own right. Low social status, people feeling less worthy or even excluded are all factors that contribute to the overall health and welfare of society at large. Therefore, the aim of policy making should be to prevent people feeling excluded or divided.

As referred to earlier, a popular misconception in tackling poverty is the assumption that once a basic minimum in material standards is attained, the causal relationship between health and poverty weakens and continues to the point of non-existence as an individual's wealth increases. However, the crucial point of the relationship between health and poverty is how relative a person's wealth is to the rest of society. Simply giving money to the less well-off is not the way to achieve this, the results of which can be seen in contemporary society, which has had the benefits of the welfare system. Increasing individual wealth and reducing the disparity between socio-economic groups can go together. Another important point is the approach there has been in the past to dealing with health. The thrust behind the development of the NHS was to treat and manage disease and ill health, which remained the focus of the NHS until recent years. Clearly, ill health and disease will remain a part of society, but new approaches to treat and prevent disease and disability need to be considered. Social relationships have been identified as providing support and giving a sense of meaning to life. A direct link has also been shown between social connectedness and morbidity. The quantity and quality of social relationships shows a direct correlation with improved health status. Therefore to reduce inequalities in health through social isolation and the breakdown of social cohesion, it is important to concentrate on community-based efforts that prevent further social disintegration and promote community growth. Berkman (1995) suggests that policy development should focus on: family-friendly work policies; statutory parental leave and the provision of quality adult and child day care; urban regeneration and development; housing policies that ensure quality accommodation regardless of income. In addition to social support, income inequality needs to be reduced. This is a hard commitment to ride as the tax and spend policies of political parties are seen as crucial to the success of a campaign election and time in government. The introduction of policies is not a 'quick fix' solution and requires time for the intended improvements and benefits to be seen. As the evidence shows, reducing income inequality is not achieved by giving more money to the poor. It is about using fiscal policies that do not penalise low wage earners, but rather support and improve low-income individuals and families.

Conclusion

Alongside long-term initiatives, such as those arising from the Social Exclusion Unit, more immediate support and intervention is needed for people experiencing poor social and health standards. For example, a person who is homeless is unlikely to have the interest or the capacity to become involved in local regeneration projects when he or she has more immediate needs such as finding a place to call home or accessing appropriate health care services for any immediate health needs. Therefore it is important that with the long-term development of public health, immediate health and social needs are not forgotten and that a balance is found. This is where the concept of partnership is very important because as a person's more immediate needs are met, they are more likely to be able to think about their future. Through partnership support of the many different health, social and voluntary services available, people are able to become part of mainstream society.

At the level of professional practice, an understanding and awareness of the concept of vulnerability is important where people are unable to advocate for themselves. This is partly the citizen advocacy as espoused by Wolfensberger (1987) who suggests that all vulnerable people need an independent advocate when coming into contact with any of the human services. In reviewing the literature, it is clear which members of society are likely to be vulnerable because of their personal and social circumstances. Essentially, those that are considered to be vulnerable members of society, are those that find themselves on the social periphery because, for one reason or another, they are unable to live within the norms set by mainstream society. Consequently, they are at risk of experiencing poor health and further social disenfranchisement. How British Society deals with that may well be how our level of civilisation is measured by history.

References

Antonovsky, A. (1987) The salutogenic perspective. Toward a new vision of health and illness. *Advances*, 4, 1, 47–55.

Appleton, J.V. (1994) The concept of vulnerability in relation to child protection: health visitors' perceptions. *Journal of Advanced Nursing*, 20, 167–75.

Berkman, L.F. (1995) The role of social relations in health. *Psychosomatic Medicine*, 57, 245–54.

Berkman, L.F. and Syme, S.L. (1979) Social Networks, host resistance and mortality: a nine-year follow-up study of Alameda County residents. *American Journal of Epidemiology*, 116, 684–94.

Big Issue (1998) *A primary health care study of vendors of the Big Issue in the North*. Manchester: Big Issue.

Black, M.E, Sheuer, M.A. and Victor, C.R. (1991) Utilisation by homeless people of acute hospital services in London. *British Medical Journal*, 301, 373–77.

Bosma, H., Marmot, M.G., Hemingway, H., Nicholson, A.G., Brunner, E. and Stansfield, A. (1997) Low job control and risk of coronary heart disease in Whitehall 11 (prospective cohort study). *British Medical Journal*, 314, 558–65.

Briggs, A. (1961) The Welfare State in historical perspective. *European Journal of Sociology*, 2, 2, 211–30.

Cassel, J. (1976) The contribution of the social environment to host resistance. *American Journal of Epidemiology*, 104, 107–23.

Cobb, S. (1976) Social support as a moderator of life stress. *Psychosomatic Medicine*, 38, 300–14.

Copp, L.A. (1986) The nurse as advocate for vulnerable persons. *Journal of Advanced Nursing*, 11, 3, 255–63.

Durkheim, E. (1951) *Suicide*. New York: Free Press.

Flaskerud, J.H. and Winslow, B.J. (1998) Conceptualising vulnerable populations: health related research. *Nursing Research*, 47, 2, 69–78.

Gilligan, J. (1996) Our Deadly Epidemic and its Causes. In Tarlov, A.R. and St Peter, R.F. (ed) (2000) *The society and population health reader: Volume II, A State and Community Perspective*. New York: The New Press.

Gordon, D., Townsend, P., Levitas, R., Pantazis, C., Payne, S., Patsios, D., Middleton, S., Ashworth, K., Adelman, L., Bradshaw, J., Williams, J. and Bramley, G. (2000) *Poverty and Social Exclusion in Britain*. York: Joseph Rowntree Foundation.

Gosling, A., Johnson, P., McCrae, J. and Paull, G. (1997) *The dynamics of low pay and unemployment in early 1990s.* London: Institute for Fiscal Studies.

Grenier, P. (1996) *Still dying for a home? An update of sick to death of homelessness.* London: Crisis.

House, J.F. (1981) *Work, Stress and Social Support.* Reading MA: Addison Wesley.

House, J.S., Landis, K.R. and Umberson, D. (1988) Social relationships and health. *Science*, 214, 186–204.

Kaplan, G., Pamuk, E., Lynch, J.W., Cohen, R.D. and Balfour, J.L. (1996) Inequality in income and mortality in the United States: analysis of mortality and potential pathways. *British Medical Journal*, 312, 999–1003.

North, C., Moore, H. and Owens, C. (1996) Go home and rest? The use of accident and emergency departments by homeless people. London: Shelter.

Philips, C.A. (1992) Vulnerability in family systems: Application to antepartum. *Journal of Perinatal and Neonatal Nursing*, 6, 3, 37–46.

Piachaud, D. (1981) Townsend and the Holy Grail. *New Society*, 421, September.

Putnam, R.D., Leonardi, R. and Nanetti, R.Y. (1993) Making Democracy Work. Civic Traditions in Modern Italy. In Kawachi, I., Kennedy, B.P. and Wilkinson, R.G. (eds) (1999) *The society and population health reader: Volume 1 Income inequality and health.* New York: The New Press.

Quick, A and Wilkinson, R.G. (1991) *Income and health.* London: Socialist Health Association.

Rogers, A.C. (1997) Vulnerability, health and health care. *Journal of Advanced Nursing*, 26, 65–72.

Rose, M.H. and Killien, M. (1983) Risk and vulnerability: A case for differentiation between personal and environmental factors that influence health and development. *Advances in Nursing Science*, 5, 3, 60–73.

Rotter, J.B. (1954) *Social Learning and Clinical Psychology.* Englewood Cliffs, NJ: Prentice-Hall.

Seeman, M. and Lewis, S. (1995) Powerlessness, Health and Mortality: A Longitudinal Study of Older Men and Mature Women. *Social Science and Medicine*, 41, 4, 517–25.

Shelter (1998) *Homelessness and health factsheet.* London: Shelter.

Spiers, J. (2000) New perspectives on vulnerability using emic and etic approaches. *Journal of Advanced Nursing*, 31, 3, 715–21.

Umberson, D. (1987) Family Health and Social Behaviours. Social control as a dimension of social integration. *Journal of Health and Social Behaviours*, 28, 3, 306–19.

United Nations (1995) *The Copenhagen declaration and programme of action: World summit for social development 6–12 March 1995.* New York: United Nations Dept. of Publications.

Victor, C.R., Connelly, J., Roderick, P. and Cohen, C. (1989) Use of hospital services by homeless families in an inner London health district. *British Medical Journal*, 299, 725–27.

Wacquant, L.J.D and Wilson, W.J. (1989) The cost of racial and class exclusion in the inner city. *Annals of the American Academy of Political and Social Science*, 501, 8–25. In Kawachi, I., Kennedy, B.P. and Wilkinson, R.G. (eds) (1999) *The society and population health reader: Volume 1 Income inequality and health.* New York: The New Press.

Wallerstein, N. (1992) Powerlessness, Empowerment and Health: Implications for Health Promotion Programs. *American Journal of Health Promotion*, 6, 3, 197–205.

Wilkinson, R.G. (1996) *Unhealthy societies. The afflictions of inequality.* London: Routledge.

Wolfensberger, W. (1987) *The New Genocide.* New York: Wolfensberger.

Further Reading

Quick, A. and Wilkinson, R.G. (1991) *Income and health.* London: Socialist Health Association.
This book is only a short read, but gives a very concise and comprehensive understanding of the relationship between income and health. It also brings together the findings of many important studies that contribute to the general consensus of opinion that income inequality adversely affects health outcomes.

Lawson, P. (1991) A home for Tom. *Nursing Times*, 87, 48, 26–9.
This is a thought-provoking article written from the author's personal experience of caring for a dying man in a hostel setting. It highlights the often complex, but very real, problems faced in caring for someone living in extraordinary social circumstances.

Rogers, A.C. (1997) Vulnerability, health and health care. *Journal of Advanced Nursing*, 26, 65–72.
This is a very informative article and lends clarity to the concept of vulnerability and how it affects a person's physiological, psychological and social functioning. It also discusses the relationship of vulnerability with a person's internal and external resources and how these resources may be used to counterbalance the effects of vulnerability.

Strehlow, A.J. and Amos-Jones, T. (1999) The homeless as a vulnerable population. *Nursing Clinics of North America*, 34, 2, 261–75.
This contributes to understanding the concept of vulnerability and its implications, with particular reference to the homeless population. It discusses the concept in relation to health and the implications this has for nursing care. It also suggests interesting policy making issues, although this is not very detailed in its examination.

6

Promoting Public Health: Media Constructions and Social Images of Health in a Post-modern Society

MARTIN KING

The key points discussed in this chapter include:

- mass media approaches to health education as part of a strategy to improve the public's health

- the need for professionals involved in public health work to note the power of media constructions of health and the way in which public perceptions of health are influenced by the media

- the lessons to be learnt from an analysis of previous health education campaigns.

Introduction

Taking a historical perspective, the chapter examines the development of mass media approaches as part of the history of public health and traces developments in different models of health education. It also argues for applying the strategies of media and cultural studies to the field of public health to make an analysis of these developments and determine the lessons we can usefully learn from this.

There have been a number of attempts over the past four decades to develop public health messages through mass media constructions. However, these are not always effective and have reflected social and political ideologies of the time. This chapter highlights the view that professionals involved in public health work need to note the power of media constructions of health and the way in which public perceptions of health are influenced by the media. They also need to make an analysis of the successes and failures of past media-based public health campaigns, paying particular attention to their origins and aims.

Using two case studies based around public information films dating from the 1940s to the 1980s, an analysis of the content, themes and approaches of the films is made. Their relationship to models of health education within a public health framework is also examined.

Finally, the chapter explores the lessons to be learned from considering or reviewing these texts together with some of the barriers which preclude them from being considered as important documents.

Professionals involved in improving public health, I would argue, need to give this twentieth century phenomenon a closer look in order to discover the potential for improving public health in the twenty-first century.

Mass Media and Health

The role of the mass media in modern society is well documented elsewhere (McCluhan, 1964; Fiske, 1987; Boyd-Barrett and Newbold, 1995). This chapter focuses primarily on television and film as media for health information. Fiske (1987) states:

> Television as – culture is a crucial part of the social dynamics by which the social structure maintains itself in a constant process of production and reproduction: meanings, population, pleasures, and their circulation are therefore part and parcel of this social structure.
>
> Television, its newness and the ways it functions in society are so multifunctional that no tightly focused theoretical perspective can provide us with adequate insight. (p. 1)

This raises some key issues concerning the academic debate about the role and influence of the mass media and its influence on the audience (McCluhan, 1964; Morley, 1980; Fiske, 1987). Here I will take an approach which attempts to explore 'How television makes, or attempts to make, meanings that serve the dominant interests in society' (Fiske, 1987:1). It is within this framework that I will examine attempts to influence and improve public health through mass media techniques with particular reference to the concepts of behaviour regulation (Lupton, 1993; Peterson, 1994) and surveillance (Armstrong, 1983; Bunton *et al.*, 1995) which I would argue have a particular relevance here. Lupton (1993), for example, talks about the way in which HIV education campaigns go beyond the factual, and contain elements of morality and lay down good and bad behaviours in relation to HIV.

Applying the analytical tools of media and cultural studies to the field of public health is a relatively recent phenomenon (Peterson, 1994; King and Watson, 2001) but a practice which many would argue is illuminative, even essential, particularly in relation to mass media campaigns.

Southwell (2000) in discussing the discourse of public health interventions states that 'in so far as such realisations are worthwhile, analysis in this vein is not idle perusal of arcane documents, but rather vital work for public health researchers' (Southwell, 2000:371). This assertion that we need to look at the way health is presented in the mass media in order to understand how the public's perceptions about health and healthy behaviours has been taken up by several authors in the field of public health. Bunton (1997), for example, in looking at contrasting representations of health in magazines from the 1950s and 1990s, argues that 'Magazines and the media are sites of increasing importance to contemporary problemalisation of health' (p. 232).

Recent work outlines the importance of examining representations of health in the mass media as part of a wider study of health and suggests 'Rather than viewing cultural studies as a discrete discipline with fixed boundaries, we would advocate the use of the strategies associated with cultural studies to interrogate "health" issues mediated by the discursive intersections of film, painting, advertising etc' (King and Watson, 2001:405). While the bringing together of media and cultural studies and public health is a relatively new idea, a long history of work on public health and health education and the mass media exists (Gatherer *et al.*, 1979; Tones, 1985).

Mass Media and Public Health

Health education as part of a public health approach can be traced back to the sanitary ladies of the 1920s, the forerunners of today's health visitors or public health nurses (Ashton and Seymour, 1988; Baggot, 2000). It is interesting to note that this approach ran alongside the structural public health reforms (see Chapter 1) rather than in isolation. The failure of the isolationist approach has been well documented over a number of decades (Hyman and Shearsley, 1947; Research Unit in Health and Behaviour Change, 1989). Baggaley (1991) states:

> Past experience with public health campaigns suggests that the mass media in isolation have little effect on health related behaviour and have to be combined with other elements for a campaign to be successful. (p. 24)

For example, the Stanford Three Community Project in the USA in the 1970s (Davis, 1987) showed how a mass media intervention over a short period of time, supported by face to face intervention methods, achieved a greater reduction in coronary heart disease risk score than media intervention alone. Similar results were found in the Finnish North Karelia Study (Koselka *et al.*, 1976). Despite this, the use of mass media techniques via print and visual media on their own has a long history of popular usage within a public health context. We tend to think of this as dating back to the 1980s with the introduction of the term health promotion (Naidoo and Wills, 1994) following the Lalonde Report (1974) and the Ottawa Charter (WHO, 1986). However, as Baggaley (1991) reveals, the use of film as a medium for health education was a development contemporary to the work of the Sanitary Ladies. 'In 1921 film was in its infancy. However, it was already apparent that the new medium held great promise for the mass communication of facts' (p. 24).

Discussion about the use of marketing and advertising techniques (McCron and Budd, 1981; Tones, 1985; Lefebvre, 1992) is a more recent phenomenon. At the heart of this debate is the question of whether mass media approaches to public health can actually change behaviour or whether they are limited to awareness raising (Ewles and Simnett, 1995; Naidoo and Wills, 1994). However, advice from the field of advertising was available as far back as 1948 with statements such as: 'Advertising is typically directed towards the canalising of pre-existing behaviours and patterns or attitudes. It seldom seeks to instil new attitudes or to create significantly new behaviour patterns' (Lazarsfield and Merton, 1948:59). This would tend to support more recent studies which point to the limitations of health education through the mass media in changing attitudes and behaviour (Tones, 1985; Redman *et al.*, 1990; Wallack *et al.*, 1993) while acknowledging its power to disseminate knowledge, raise awareness and place public health issues on the public agenda.

As health education developed as part of the public health movement at the beginning of the twentieth century it drew heavily on models borrowed from psychology, initially employing very simplistic knowledge – practice approaches (Bennett and Murphy, 1997), which assumed that a change in knowledge levels would lead directly to behaviour change. This is important to remember when considering the case studies later in this chapter.

This emphasis on models continued up until the 1980s. Models such as the Health Belief Model (Becker, 1974); The Health Action Model (Tones *et al.*, 1990); The Theory of Reasoned Action (Azjen and Fishbein, 1980) and The Theory of Planned Behaviour (Azjen, 1988) provided a theoretical framework for health education campaigns, particularly those conducted via the mass media. Thus, the focus of these social-cognition models is on individual behaviour or the individual in relation to their environment:

> Social cognition models ... provide a parsimonious understanding of the cognitive processes involved in behavioural decision making. Behaviour is considered conse-quent to a complex process of involving consideration of attitudes, cost-benefit analysis, and outcomes and efficacy judgements. While the emphasis of the model is on cognitive factors, social and environmental processes are also considered in the form of social norms, barriers to change and in Azjen's dimension of control over behaviour. (Bennett and Murphy, 1997:43)

So far, then, we have established that public health practitioners have a wealth of research evidence about models of behaviour change, and the role of the mass media in this process, available to them. However, I would argue that this evidence has not always been best utilised. For example, what we see from the 1960s onwards is an emphasis on behav-iour and life-style as the cause of ill health; an emphasis which ignores what we know about the development of the public health movement in the UK (see Chapter 1). This can be illustrated by government responses to the fact that no inroads were being made into the big killers, for exam-ple, CHD and cancer, despite post-war prosperity and the success of the NHS (Ashton and Seymour, 1988).

The publication of *Prevention and Health: Everybody's Business* (DHSS, 1976) is seen as the epitome of the life-style approach. This emphasis on behaviour and life-style is reiterated in *Promoting Better Health* (DHSS, 1987a) and reappears again in *The Health of the Nation* (DoH, 1992). However, following the publication of the *Targets for Health* (WHO, 1985) new systems models of health education began to develop which, follow-ing in the footsteps of the Lalonde Report (1974) and the Ottawa Charter (WHO, 1986), perceived health as the result of the interaction of a number of factors including socio-economic status, environment, class and gender, as well as behaviour. It can be argued that this marked a return to a holis-tic public health approach akin to that of the nineteenth-century reform-ers, which eventually spawned the terms health promotion and the new public health. (Naidoo and Wills, 1994, Chapter 4, provide a useful review of the development of Health Education and Health Promotion.) Models developed by Beattie (1991) and Seedhouse (1997) are also good examples of this holistic approach.

However, while academics and practitioners may have shifted their views, it is worth noting that politicians had not. A Tory government committed to an ideology of individualism (Hall, 1988) abolished the Health Education Council in the 1980s and replaced it with the less inde-pendent Health Education Authority. This followed a dispute between the Chief Executive of the Health Education Council, David Player, and the Government over comments he had made about the role of the alcohol and tobacco industries and their contribution to increasing ill health (Naidoo and Wills, 1994). This conflict between political/ideological agendas and academic/practitioner knowledge/experience helps to explain why the history of public health in the UK reflects a combination of individualistic, life-style based approaches and wider attempts at socioeconomic engineering.

It is against this backdrop that health education in the mass media must be considered. As we have already seen, historically, mass media health education has had a recognised role in the public health movement. The criticisms and limitations outlined previously, combined with the emergence of the new public health movement (Ashton and Seymour, 1988), with its emphasis on changing environments, marked the end of an era. Widespread use of film and TV to encourage behaviour conducive to improving the public's health began to decline. The use of public information films, especially popular from the 1940s to the 1970s, have now declined to the point where only the seasonal drink–drive ads and the occasional anti-smoking campaign remain, to remind us of this particular aspect of health education. The much criticised AIDS campaigns of the late 1980s (Wellings, 1988; Wober, 1988; HEA, 1992) seemed to mark the death knell for this genre.

Emerging work on resistance to health education messages (Crossley, 2001) can be combined with previously discussed studies on the regulatory power of the media (Bell, 1992; Lupton, 1993; Peterson, 1994) and criticism of mass media health education (McCron and Budd, 1981; McGuire, 1992; Egger *et al.*, 1993) to provide an explanation. However, the eternal question of whether we have thrown the baby out with the bath water is pertinent here. To illustrate this a case study approach will now be taken. Using public information films from the 1940s to the 1980s, an attempt will be made to map them against developments in approaches to improving public health, explore content and themes and examine their re-presentation to a contemporary audience via television. This raises issues around lessons to be learned about using health education in the mass media as part of a public health strategy, and provides examples which employ a variety of approaches.

Case Studies

The case studies which follow have been analysed within a documentary research framework:

> There are a wide variety of documentary sources at our disposal for social research. Documents inform the practical and political decisions which people make on

a daily and long term basis and many even construct a particular reading of past social or political events. They can tell us about the aspirations and intentions of the period to which they refer and describe places and social relationships at a time when we may not have been born, or were simply not present. (May, 1993:133)

Some of the tools and techniques developed as part of the disciplines of research methods and media and cultural studies have been used to examine public health texts from a specific era. These include content analysis (Robson, 1993) and critical discourse analysis (Chouliraki and Fairclough, 1999). These methods allow us to examine or excavate texts (books, magazines, articles, films) to look more closely at the use of language and imagery and together with their intended or unintended meanings.

Case Study 1 – Charley Says

Charley Says is a collection of animated public information films ranging from 1959 to 1983. This 'text' is chosen for a number of reasons. First it is an accessible collection of popular public information films and provides examples for analysis in the light of the previous debate, that is the use of health education in the mass media as part of a wider public health strategy. Second, they are being re-presented as nostalgic entertainment, marketed as 'The best public information films in the world Volume 1'.

> Public Information Films were as much a part of the 70s culture as tank tops, platform shoes and the Bay City Rollers. Now you can relive the age of bad taste and dodgy hairdos, with this collection of the most memorable animated Public Information Films provided by the Central Office of Information. (*Network/Sound and Media*, 1998)

Marketed rather falsely, as part of the late 1990s 70s retro boom (given that they range from the 1950s to the 1980s) the collection is offered as entertainment, a look back (with humour?) at the past, a theme that will be explored further in the second case study. What the collection does offer is an opportunity to examine the range of health topics that were seen to be important to the public in order to improve public health. Topics covered include: road safety (*Rude on the Road*, 1959); the environment (*When in the Country*, 1963); home safety (*Tidy up at Night*, 1969); child safety (*Tell Mummy*, 1969); water safety (*Iced Ponds*, 1969); careers (*Jobs for Young Girls*, 1970); safety at work (*Lifting Safely*, 1972); nuclear attack (*Protect and Survive – Action After Warnings/Causalities*, 1975) and travel advice (*Malaria Warning*, 1983). What is immediately striking is that this range of topics conceptualised public health in a broad way. Health is about the environment (water supplies, the countryside), legislation (health and safety) and war (nuclear attack) as well as behaviours (on the road, in the home, around water). Interestingly, this approach to public health has more in common with the nineteenth-century public health reforms and the new public health movement of the 1990s than the life-style approaches popular at the time they were made.

This again draws our attention to the issue of political versus practitioner agendas. The range of topics covered in the public information films is much broader in scope and certainly conceptualises health in a much broader sense than the examples of health education in the mass media which replaced the public information film genre. For example, the AIDS adverts of the 1980s (HEA, 1992), the heroin campaigns of the 1980s (DHSS, 1987b) and the subsequent sporadic campaigns around smoking (McGuire, 1992), all focus on individual behaviours around particular diseases. While there is an element of this in public information films, which often tread a fine line between attempts at awareness raising and behaviour change, disease-based topics are notable by their absence (smoking for example). The topics covered here would sit comfortably within Seedhouse's foundations model of health (Seedhouse, 1997) with its conceptualisation of health based on a broad hierarchy of needs, first developed by Maslow (1973). Seedhouse argues that public health work must focus on meeting basic needs first – food, shelter, warmth, education – before progressing to interventions which address specific illnesses and associated behaviours.

I would also argue that, as the films in the collection progress from the 1960s to the 1980s, a change in approach can be traced from a gentle, light, humorous, awareness raising to a darker, accusing, victim-blaming approach (Ewles and Simnett, 1995; Naidoo and Wills, 1994). These assertions will be illustrated by the following examples.

When in the Country (1963) provides a good example of the genre of this period. Rather than attempting to change behaviour with one short sharp message, the film provides four minutes of awareness raising around countryside and environmental issues conceptualised as public health issues, with a range of topics being incorporated. Presented in cartoon format the film draws on contemporary colours and stylised drawings to the accompaniment of a jazz soundtrack, all of which creates an atmosphere of entertainment as well as information. This is what Moynihan (1995) describes as the use of heuristic or positive appeals – the creation of a positive, appealing environment in which to present the message.

The key theme of showing consideration for others, which is apparent in a number of other films in the collection (*Rude on the Road*, 1959 – a plea for courtesy and consideration for other road users and pedestrians; *Safeguarding Water Supplies*, 1965 – information on how to keep streams and rivers unpolluted), represents a communitarian approach which is a major feature of many of these early examples. Etzioni's (1995) work on a return to communitarian values and his work on rights and responsibilities has informed the present Government's approach to welfare reform. His influential work calls for a return to a sense of community, a backlash against the individualistic, anti-society ideology of right-wing governments in the US and UK in the 1980s. He sets out this communitarian thesis as follows:

The Communitarian Movement – which is an environmental movement dedicated to the betterment of our moral, social and political environment – seeks to sort out these principles. And Communitarians are dedicated to working with our fellow citizens to bring about the changes in values, habits and public policies that will allow us to do for society what the environmental movement seeks to do for nature: to safeguard and enhance our future. (Etzioni, 1995:3)

In *When in the Country* we are asked to be considerate to the farmer (park with consideration – the townie E-Type Jaguar owner parking across an entrance to a field); leave the farmers things alone (don't mess with machinery); to animals in the countryside (train your dog to obey you, let birds and wild animals live their lives undisturbed); to the environment (trees are valuable as well as beautiful); keep fire under control, and to generally behave like good citizens. Again, citizenship is a key concept of Etzioni's (1995) work which attempts to draw on ideas about community which pre-date the new right, individualistic approaches to health and welfare of the 1980s (Hall, 1988).

This gentle, complex, humorous, informative awareness-raising approach from 1963 can be contrasted with a similar 'follow the country code' film from 1971 (*Joe and Petunia – Country Code*). Featuring Joe and Petunia, popular characters in the collection, as a working class couple not knowing how to behave in the country. The couple are depicted leaving litter, letting their dog run wild, trampling on crops and leaving gates open. The short film (62 seconds) ends with an angry red-faced farmer hopping up and down saying, 'When folk come out to the country, why, oh why, won't they follow the Country Code?'. The tone of the film is more direct, confrontational and victim blaming – bad behaviours are also exhibited and confrontation ensues.

In a similar way we can contrast the approaches of *Iced Ponds* (1969) with *Frozen Ponds* (1980). Both warn of the dangers of skating on frozen ponds – perhaps a quaint notion today, but at the time it was seen as a topic worthy of inclusion in the public information film repertoire. *Iced Ponds* features stylised cartoon graphics similar to those of *When in the Country*. Its overall feel is light – the white background predominates and the sun features in several scenes. Ten children (communitarian theme) take an old man and throw him on to the ice to test it – the atmosphere is humorous and upbeat, that is, this can be fun and safe, with the three key safety messages repeated: take an adult; wait until the ice has been tested; and keep away from the edge. End message – as a result they lived happily ever after!

By way of contrast *Frozen Ponds* (1980) has a dark shadowy backdrop of black, purple and yellow, and ends with a night scene. With the use of cartoon graphics the drawings are realistic. The voice-over is in the form of a police officer at the scene of an accident at a frozen pond, radioing details back to the station ('It was getting dark before they found him, Sir'). A body is being put into an ambulance, the flashing light providing an eerie backdrop. Someone is to blame – the message is gendered (Tyler, 1995; Hooks, 1997). The blame falls on the mother ('She said she never dreamed that it was dangerous'). This dark, individualistic victim-blaming approach with its use of fear appeals (Severin and Tankard, 1989) is a forerunner of the approaches that would be used in AIDS and drug campaigns later in the decade (DHSS, 1987b; Wober, 1988).

A number of issues raised in these films will be drawn together by way of conclusions on these at the end of the chapter.

Case Study 2 – You Don't Want to Do That!

This second case study is a 40-minute programme produced in 2001 by the BBC entitled *You don't want to do that* (BBC, 2001a) – a title borrowed from the catchphrase of one of comedian Harry Enfield's creations (BBC, 1996). The character in question offers advice on the best way to carry out certain activities and on what not to do; hence its relevance to a show which takes a humorous look at clips of public information films of the 1950s, 1960s and 1970s. The programme is illuminative, in that it explores themes around the past–present relationship (*Popular Memory Group*, 1982) in which a binary opposition (Levi-Strauss, 1968) is set up. Past equates to bad, amusing, naïve and present equates to good, serious, common-sense (Gramsci, 1971; Geertz, 1983).

The format is an increasingly popular one for the BBC; other examples include *Before they were famous* (BBC, 2001c) presented by Angus Deaton, in which the audience is invited to laugh at the fact that famous people were once in either less famous shows/films or less famous/glamorous roles, via a series of clips. *TV's finest failures* (BBC, 2001b), presented by Phil Jupitas, invites the audience to laugh at bad-quality or failed programmes from the previous decades. The irony is that these shows represent low-budget, poor-quality formula TV; invited audiences, garish set, c-list celebrity host presenting a series of clips from previous decades to amuse the TV audience. I would argue that the concepts of surveillance (Nettleton, 1992) and regulation (Foucault, 1980) previously discussed in the context of public information films can also be applied to this genre of TV programming and in particular specifically to this case study.

There is a strategy of containment (Fiske, 1987) at work in which the audience are directed by the hosts and respond appropriately. The raw clip is cooked (Levi-Strauss, 1968) by the host's linking dialogue in order to make sense of it for the audience. A selective version of reality is offered by the host. Rather than allowing the audience to examine the raw film clips on offer, to decide on their meanings and draw conclusions, the format of the show (recognised by the audience) is designed merely to use these interesting 'texts' as the butt of a series of jokes.

> 'The truth' only exists in the studio, yet that 'truth' depends for its authenticity upon the actuality film, those pieces of 'raw reality' whose meanings are actually made by the discourse of the studio. (Fiske, 1987:288–9)

The host chosen for *You don't want to do that* is Jeremy Clarkson, former host of the testosterone-charged *Top Gear* (BBC, 1978–present) and well known for his politically incorrect views and no nonsense approach to TV presenting. These personal traits are important in setting the tone. Analysis of the text (scripted by comedian Danny Baker) provides us with a clue as to what version of the truth (past – bad, naïve, stupid) is at work here. I would contend that Fiske's (1987) work on news is useful here with the host (Clarkson in this case) performing the same function as a newsreader in constructing a particular version of the truth.

> The central space is that of the studio newsreader, who does not appear to be author of his/her own discourse, but who speaks the objective discourse of 'the truth'. Paradoxically, the newsreader's personal traits, such as reliability or credibility, are often used to undermine the objectivity of the discourse. (Fiske, 1987:288)

Clarkson's introduction conceptualises the 'truth' about the public information films we, the audience, are about to see and sets the theme for the linking texts of the programme. 'Together over the next forty minutes, we're going to take an astounded [*sic*] look at that branch of the broadcasting industry that exists only to tell you off. It's the kind of state-backed initiative that believes you're a fool or a nincompoop' (BBC, 2001a).

Thus the critical literature on health education via the mass media is summarised for popular consumption. The audience is drawn into the anti-state philosophy of Clarkson's truth by subtle flattery, that is, of course we are not fools or nincompoops. This is a good example of what Geertz (1983), developing Gramsci's (1971) theory of hegemony, describes as the use of common-sense approaches in the media – the way in which ideas are presented as common sense and unchallengeable. In this example, Clarkson's labelling of public information films as part of a 'nanny-state' is a political and ideological stance disguised as 'common sense', or that which goes without saying. As Geertz states:

> As a frame of a thought, and a species of it, commonsense is as totalising as any other: no religion is more dogmatic, no science more ambitious, no philosophy more general. Its tonalities are different and so are the arguments to which it appeals, but like them – and like art and like ideology, it pretends to reach past illusion to truth, to, as we say, things as they are. (Geertz, 1983:84)

What Barthes (1973) calls 'ex-nomination' is at work here. 'That which is ex-nominated appears to have no ulterior motive and is thus granted the status of the rational, the universal, or that-which-cannot-be-challenged' (Fiske, 1987:290). The anti-fun nature of public information films is then tackled. 'You've got some TV that wants to have fun and games and then this sort that brings along a note to say it has a runny nose. And, what's more, it says that you mustn't have fun either' (BBC, 2001a).

A link is then made to more contemporary the no-fun TV – *Watchdog* with Lyn Faulds-Wood (BBC, 1985–present) part of the consumer culture (Featherstone, 1991; Baudrillard, 1998) TV which followed in the wake of Esther Rantzen's *That's Life* (BBC, 1974–1994). Faulds-Wood is described as the all-powerful nanny, the queen of questions, the party-pooping empress of interference. The terms 'nanny' and 'interference' are of course redolent of the writings of those who were part of the Thatcherite New Right, individualistic ideology of the 1970s and 1980s (Hall, 1988). Further analysis uncovers a particular view of gender (Tyler, 1995; Hooks, 1997) and behaviour: 'My guess is that while we are all growing up hooked on *Grandstand*, *Top of the Pops* and *Catweazle*, Lyn was studying the work that went into such essential warnings as this' (BBC, 2001a) (cut to clip of *The Fatal Floor*, 1974 – a film about the dangers of putting rugs on to polished floors).

The 'female' 'nanny' and 'queen' of party pooping contrasts with the 'masculine' *Grandstand* and fun-filled *Top of the Pops* (plus an excellent obscure left field reference to *Catweazle*). The common-sense (Geertz, 1983) notion of healthy and unhealthy interests is also implied in this piece of text.

Finally, in terms of looking at the linking text, the past–present relationship emerges as a passing theme, but with no real analysis or exploration of the issues raised. Following the clip of *The Fatal Floor*, Clarkson states: 'such slices of alarmist finger wagging were as common on TV in the 60s and 70s as gardening and makeover programmes are today' (BBC, 2001a). He then asks the question 'Who woke up one morning and thought "I know what I'll do today, I'll make a film about the perils of loose rugs on shiny surfaces?" ' (BBC, 2001a). Here, interestingly, the dominant discourse is rooted in the previously discussed binary oppositions of past bad – present good.

Clarkson *could* easily have examined the previous two statements by asking an equally valid question: 'Who woke up one morning and thought "I know what I'll do today, I'll make an endless series of formulaic, repetitive programmes in which the audience watches people decorating and doing the gardening?" ' However, to do so would be to undermine the astounded [*sic*] view the audience have been invited to take of the past in the programme's introduction. We are laughing at the past here – not analysing the present. No dissenting voices are allowed (Hall, 1980; Fiske, 1987; Hooks, 1997) and the 'common-sense' view presented by Clarkson predominates. The idea that TV viewers of the 1960s and 1970s might have been astounded to see decorating and gardening programmes in such great proliferation on prime time TV is never raised. Thus any real analysis of the relationship between past and present TV is denied. The programme falls into the comedy genre but the dominant discourse previously outlined often obscures the content of the clips themselves. It can be argued that these clips provide an interesting insight into attempts to address public health issues through the mass media and reflect a set of views and attitudes from the past which are different to those of the present.

Again, historically, it is interesting to examine the range of topics conceptualised as part of public health and public information. These include: home hygiene (*Clean food*, 1945); road safety (*How to drive*, 1964); outdoor safety (*Overhead danger*, 1979); the work of the police force (*The Blue Lamp*, 1966). More traditional health education topics are also included: seat belt safety (*Clunk Click*, 1977); crossing the road (*Tufty and Friends*, 1973). Also, in this latter section (*Green Cross Code*, 1974) we are invited by the host (within the past–present binary framework) to be amused by the personalities used in the films – footballer Kevin Keegan, singers Alvin Stardust and Les Gray (of MUD) and boxer Joe

Bugner, as well as by their insane and uncoordinated clothing. The opportunity to examine the interesting use of contemporary role models as part of an approach to road safety
education is passed over in favour of a joke about huge flares and kipper ties.

Summarising this section, I would advance the view that there is further
work to be done on audience reaction to public information films and on
memory and retention of messages. I would contend that this may be a
useful avenue to explore in determining what can be learnt from past
attempts to address public health issues through the mass media, and how
they can in fact inform present thinking. The difference between the format of the two case studies – one as a straightforward presentation of clips
with nostalgia and entertainment value, the other contained and regulated
via a linking dialogue – may also be interesting to explore further when
examining the suitability of TV as a medium for what we now recognise
as a complex public health and health education message.

Conclusion

This chapter has raised a number of issues pertinent to the debate on the
use of mass media as a public health strategy. It has attempted to unravel
some of the complexities inherent in using such methods.

Past attempts exist in the form of 'texts' or 'documents' and are available
for present-day public health practitioners to examine. The introduction of
the concepts and tools of media and cultural studies into the field of
public health has been a useful step towards unravelling the successes and
failures of these past attempts. This chapter has used public information
films as an example of such attempts and there are, I would contend, some
key lessons to be learned. Not least of these is the relationship between the
past and the present – how we approach the history of public health will
determine how much we can usefully learn. Contemporary approaches,
whether the use of mass media, or other methods of education, need to be
open to criticism and based on what we can successfully learn from past
failures and successes. This in essence *is* evidence based practice.

Another key issue raised for consideration in the chapter has been what
is termed the political/ideological versus the academic/practitioner
agenda. The first part of the chapter maps theoretical developments in
concepts of 'health' and the attempts to change public health through
different approaches. However, against those developments we must also
consider the political/ideological agenda. So, for example, adverts from
the 1980s around smoking and HIV reflect an approach rooted in an individualistic approach to health education, which makes assumptions about

an individual's control over their own 'health'. This, in a period where socio-economic and environmental models of health and health related behaviour have been developed, academically and also in practice.

By way of contrast, examples of public information films from the 1950s and 1960s (*Rude on the Road, When in the Country* – outlined previously) reflect a broader conceptualisation of health and communitarian themes which seem out of step with our understanding of the predominance of individually focussed approaches to health education at that time.

It is also useful to examine the specific aims of the films. Given the limitations of mass media approaches in isolation to produce behaviour change, it is useful to distinguish between attempts at behaviour change and awareness raising and fear appeal approaches, or those which appear to lay down moral and regulatory frameworks. The contrasting awareness raising and victim-blaming themes outlined in the first case study provide a good example of these different approaches. By this sort of examination we can start to learn something useful about the use of mass media methods in public health and to raise questions about the fall in its popularity. There is, however, further work to be done in this area.

Finally, what seems striking when watching these films is the focus on contemporary public health issues. Above and beyond what they might reveal about conceptualisation of health and methodological approaches, many of the issues covered are still regarded as key areas of public health work. Courtesy on the road, child safety and stranger danger, road traffic accidents and the town/countryside debate are just four key contemporary areas which are addressed in this historical collection.

Given that the power and influence of the mass media in modern society shows no signs of abating, awareness raising and education through mass media approaches still have a role to play in addressing modern-day public health issues. The key to the future success of such approaches lies in the lessons learnt from the past.

References

Armstrong, D. (1983) *Political Anatomy of the Body: Medical Knowledge in Britain in the 20th Century.* Cambridge: Cambridge University Press.

Ashton, J. and Seymour, H. (1988) *The New Public Health.* Buckingham: Open University Press.

Azjen, I. and Fishbein, M. (1980) *Understanding Attitudes and Predicting Behaviour.* Englewood Cliffs, NJ: Prentice-Hall.

Azjen, I. (1988) *Attitudes, Personality and Behaviour.* Buckingham: Open University Press.

Baggaley, J. (1991) Media Health Campaigns: not just what you say, but the way you say it. In *WHO – AIDS Prevention through Health Promotion* facing sensitive issues. Amsterdam: World Health Organisation.

Baggot, R. (2000) *Public Health, Policy and Politics.* London: Macmillan.

Barthes, R. (1973) *Mythologies.* London: Paladin.

Baudrillard, J. (1998) *The Consumer Society: Myths and Structures*. London: Sage.

BBC TV (1974–1994) *That's Life*. BBC.

BBC TV (1978–present) *Top Gear*. BBC.

BBC TV (1985–present) *Watchdog*. BBC.

BBC TV (1996) *Harry Enfield's Television Programme*. Series 2, Part 1, BBC TV, radio, video.

BBC TV (2001a) *You Don't Want To Do That*. BBC 1, 11.2.01, at 21.20.

BBC TV (2001b) *Before they were famous*. BBC1, 24.8.01, at 21.20.

BBC TV (2001c) *TV's Finest Failures*. BBC, 19.10.01, at 23.05.

Beattie, A. (1991) Knowledge and Control in Health Promotion: a test case for social policy and social theory. In Gabe, J., Calnan, M. and Bury, M. (eds) *The Sociology of the Health Service*. London: Routledge.

Becker, M.H. (1974) The Health Belief Model and Personal Health Behaviour. *Health Education Monographs*, 2, 324–508.

Bell, P. (1992) *Multicultural Australia in the Media. A report to the Office of Multicultural Affairs*. Canberra: ACPS.

Bennett, P. and Murphy, P. (1997) *Psychology and Health Promotion*. Buckingham: Open University Press.

Boyd-Barrett, O. and Newbold, C. (1995) *Approaches to Media. A Reader*. London: Routledge.

Bunton, R. (1997) Popular Health, Advanced Liberalism and Good Housekeeping Magazine. In Peterson, A. and Bunton, R. (eds) *Foucault, Health and Medicine*, 223–48, London: Routledge.

Bunton, R., Nettleton, S. and Burrows, R. (eds) (1995) *The Sociology of Health Promotion. Critical Analyses of Consumption, Life-style and Risks*. London: Routledge.

Chouliraki, L. and Fairclough, N. (1999) *Critical Discourse Analysis – the Critical Study of Language*. London: Longman.

Crossley, M. (2001) 'Resistance' and Health Promotion. *Health Education Journal*, 60, 3, 197–204.

Davis, A.M. (1987) Heart Health Campaigns. *Health Education Journal*, 39, 74–9.

DHSS (Department of Health and Social Security) (1976) *Prevention and Health: Everybody's Business*. London: HMSO.

DHSS (Department of Health and Social Security) (1987a) *Promoting Better Health*. London: HMSO.

DHSS (Department of Health and Social Security) (1987b) *Anti Heroin Campaign. Stage 5 Research Evaluation*. London: DHSS.

DoH (Department of Health) (1992) *The Health of the Nation*. London: HMSO.

Egger, G., Donovan, R. and Spark, R. (1993) *Health and the Media: Principles and Practice for Health Promotion*. Sydney: McGraw-Hill.

Etzioni, A (1995) *The Spirit of Community*. London: Fontana Press.

Ewles, L. and Simnett, I. (1995) *Promoting Health. A Practical Guide*. London: Scutari Press.

Featherstone, M. (1991) *Consumer Culture and Post Modernism*. London: Sage.

Fiske, J. (1987) *Television Culture*. London: Routledge.

Foucault, M. (1980) *Power/Knowledge*. New York: Pantheon.

Gatherer, A., Parfit, J., Parker, E. and Vessey, M. (1979) *Is Health Education Effective?* London: Health Education Council.

Geertz, C. (1983) *Local Knowledge*. New York: Basic Books.

Gramsci, A. (1971) *Selections from the Prison Notebooks*. London: Lawrence and Wiseheart.

Hall, S. (1980) Encoding/Decoding. In Hall, S., Hobson, D., Lowe, A. and Willis, S.P., *Culture, Media, Language: Working Papers in Cultural Studies*, 128–38. London: Hutchinson.

Hall, S. (1988) *The Hard Road to Renewal, Thatcherism and the Crisis of the Left*. London: Verso.

HEA (Health Education Authority) (1992) *Does it Work? Perspectives on the Evaluation of HIV/AIDS Health Promotion*. London: Health Education Authority.

Hooks, B. (1997) *Reel to Reel*. London: Routledge.

Hyman, C.F. and Shearsley, P. (1947) Some reasons why information campaigns fail. *Public Opinion Quarterly*, 11, 413–23.

King, M. and Watson, K. (2001) Transgressing Venues: Health Studies, Cultural Studies and the Media. *Health Care Analysis*, 9, 4, 401–13.

Koselka, K., Puska, P. and Tuomilheto, J. (1976) The North Karelia Project. A first evaluation. *International Journal of Health Education*, 19, 59–66.

Lalonde, M. (1974) *A new perspective on the Health of Canadians*. Ottawa: Information Canada.

Lazarsfield, P.F. and Merton, R.K. (1948) Mass Communications, popular taste and organised social action. In Bryson, L. (ed.) *The Communication of Ideas*, 59–73, New York: Harper.

Lefebvre, R.C. (1992) Social Marketing and Health Promotion. In Bunton, R. and MacDonald, G. (eds) *Health Promotion, Disciplines and Diversity*. London: Routledge.

Levi-Strauss, C. (1968) *Structural Anthropology*. London: Penguin.

Lupton, D. (1993) AIDS, risk and heterosexuality in the Australian Press. *Discourse and Society*, 4, 3, 13–19.

McCluhan, M. (1964) *Understanding Media*. London: Routledge & Kegan Paul.

McCron, R. and Budd, S. (1981) The Role of the Mass Media in Health Education: an analysis. In Meyer, M. (ed.) *Health Education by television and radio*. Munich: K.G. Saur.

McGuire, C. (1992) *Pausing for Breath: A review of No Smoking Day Research, 1984–1991*. London: Health Education Authority.

Maslow, A.H., (1973) *Dominance, Self Esteem, Self Actualisation. The Germinal Papers of A.H. Maslow*. London: Sage.

May, T. (1993) *Social Research: Issues, Methods and Process*. Buckingham: Open University Press.

Morley, D. (1980) *The Nationwide Archive*. London: British Film Institute.

Moynihan, J. (1995) Thinking Positively. In Maiback, E. and Parrott, R. (eds) *Designing Health Messages*. London: Sage.

Naidoo, J. and Wills, J. (1994) *Health Promotion, Foundations for Practice*. London: Balliere Tindall.

Nettleton, S. (1992) *Power, Pain and Dentistry*. Buckingham: Open University Press.

Network/Sound and Media (1998) *Charley Says*. Network/Sound and Media: video.

Peterson, A. (1994) Governing Images. Media Construction of the 'Normal', 'Healthy' Subject. *Media Information*, Australia 72, 32–40.

Popular Memory Group (1982) *Popular Memory: Theory, Politics, Method, in Centre for Contemporary Cultural Studies, Making Histories: Studies in History, Writing and Politics*. London: Hutchinson.

Redman, S., Spencer, E. and Sanson-Fisher, W. (1990) The Role of the Mass Media in changing health related behaviour: a Critical Appraisal of two models. *Health Promotion International*, 5, 1, 85–103.

Research Unit in Health and Behaviour Change (1989) *Changing the Public Health*. Chichester: John Wiley and Sons.

Robson, C. (1993) *Real World Research – A Guide for Social Scientists and Practitioner Researchers*. Oxford: Blackwell.

Seedhouse, D. (1997) *Health Promotion: Philosophy, Prejudice and Practice*. Chichester: Wiley.

Severin, W.J. and Tankard, J.W. (1989) *Communication Theories*. London: Longman.

Southwell, B. (2000) Audience Constructions and AIDS Education Efforts: exploring communication assumptions of public health interventions. *Critical Public Health*, 10, 3, 314–9.

Tones, B.K. (1985) The use and abuse of mass media in health promotion. *Health Education Research, Theory and Practice*, pilot issue, 9–14.

Tones, K., Tilford, S. and Robinson, Y. (1990) *Health Education, Effectiveness and Efficiency*. London: Chapman and Hall.

Tyler, P. (1995) *Screening the Sexes*. New York: Da Capo.

Wallack, L., Dorforman, L., Jennigan, D. and Themba, M. (1993) *Media Advocacy and Public Health, Power for Prevention*. London: Sage.

Wellings, K. (1988) Perceptions of Risk – Media treatments of Aids. In Aggleton, P. and Homans, H. (eds) *Social Aspects of AIDS*. London: The Falmer Press.

WHO (World Health Organisation) (1985) *Targets for Health*. Geneva: WHO.

WHO (World Health Organisation) (1986) *Ottawa Charter*. Geneva: WHO.

Wober, J.M. (1988) Informing the British Public about AIDS. *Health Education Research*, 3, 19–24.

Part III

The Professionalisation of Public Health: Current and Future Perspectives

Chapters 7, 8 and 9 are designed to enable the reader to look at the way public health is currently assessed and measured in contemporary society and the way government responses shape the way social issues are managed by health care professionals. Chapter 7 illustrates the social diversity of need as well as the problems associated with providing public health services to those who are often at the periphery of society and whose needs are the most difficult to meet. This chapter identifies how, using a narrative approach, individuals can be given a voice to express their health needs. Chapter 8 focuses on social exclusion and the work of the Government's Social Exclusion Units (SEUs), critically examining political responses to public health and considering how far political change has influenced the fundamental problem of social inequality. Individual case studies highlight different social needs and are used to illustrate the processes involved in social exclusion. The final chapter reflects on previous chapters and emphasises the key themes and issues highlighted throughout the book. The chapter explores the professional response to public health ultimately assessing the role of public health nursing for improving health. The chapter expands current thinking on public health nursing and looks at the potential for improving and developing practice in this topical area.

Part III

The Professionalisation of Public Health: Current and Future Perspectives

7

Identifying the Health Needs of Communities and Populations

MARIA HORNE

The key points discussed in this chapter include:

- health needs assessment and its development as an integral process whereby public health can respond to local and national priorities
- the concepts underpinning health, needs and assessment
- the role played by assessment of health needs in improving the health of a population.

Introduction

This chapter will critique health needs assessment as a concept and evaluate the possibilities for improving the public health through health needs assessment. Health philosophy underpins the activity of health needs assessment and the prevailing philosophy of health will have an impact on the form of needs assessment that is undertaken. Indeed much of what is discussed as health needs assessment is clearly health *care* needs assessment and is generally a way of making decisions about resource allocation. Since 1997 we have arguably witnessed a change of philosophy at governmental level which finally recognises the increasing inequalities in health (see Brocklehurst's chapter) and the broader approach to health and its improvement that needs to be taken in order to reduce them. The New Labour Government elected in 1997 certainly seem, more than any government since the National Health Service was instituted, intent on identifying the social factors that lead to the inequalities in health and pulling all public services together in working to meet the needs in order to reduce them. This has led ultimately to the drive for public health approaches that are the key features of the most recent government documents (for example DoH, 2001).

The health *care* needs assessment approach is based on epidemiological and economic perspectives of health. The epidemiological approach defines health negatively and attempts to quantify health, or rather the absence of health, in the form of mortality and morbidity rates for different diseases and deprivation indices. While this does of course identify the results of the different determinants of health, it does not identify or measure the determinants themselves. In this way, the epidemiological approach could be argued to be measuring the symptoms rather than the causes of ill health.

The economic approach views health in terms of cost, demand, utility and supply. It quantifies health through quality-adjusted life year estimates (QALYs), in an attempt to calculate costs of treatment (Bowling, 1997a). Therefore, QALYs are not measures of quality of life but measures of units of benefit from a medical intervention, reflecting change in survival with a weighting factor for quality of life (Bowling, 1997b). The main focus of this approach emphasises that, owing to limited resources, areas of need are relative and may be 'traded off' between their estimated benefits, estimated harm and costs, providing rationalisation of health service provision (Billings and Cowley, 1995). This economic approach to assessment of health needs assumes a single world view presented in a quasi-scientific way, that is the utilitarian view that the greatest good is perfect health. It is this view that undermines the good that is possible when an individual is 'imperfect' in any way and it is a view that could be argued to be a driving force behind many developed countries' service provision.

There are of course alternative world views of health and needs and taking these into account when assessing health and health need would incorporate a broader approach which for example would take into account the social and psychological dimensions of health. However, even taking into consideration these dimensions we cannot be assured that health needs assessment is all inclusive. Britain is a diverse, pluralistic and multicultural society and, as identified by Spanswick (Chapter 5) and Costello *et al.* (Chapter 4), we have not developed a sufficient level of cultural sensitivity within this country to be confident that tools of health needs assessment will encapsulate the health needs of the commonly excluded groups.

Health needs assessment has evolved from its origins as a medical tool for assessing health care needs, into a more pluralistic process of exploring, from a multiple 'voices' perspective, both health and health care needs. The literature reveals that over the years health needs assessment has been variously described as a process integral to raising consciousness (Marti-Costa and Serrano-Garcia, 1995), as well as a strategy for assessing needs (Billings, 1996). It has also been seen as a way of fulfilling need and demand for health care by populations in order to improve the effectiveness of health care delivery (Stevens and Gabbay, 1991).

Within the NHS, assessment of health needs has been seen as a requirement of purchasing and commissioning authorities (DoH, 1990). More contemporary evidence, however, suggests that it is now viewed as an integral process by which primary care can respond to local and national priorities (NHSME, 1992; DoH, 1997, 1999a). Hence, health needs assessment has a central role within contemporary health care thinking, strategy and service delivery (Billings, 1996). It is clearly a multilayered concept in that it is recognised as a way of helping planners to devise services in a more rational manner. Also, in an ideal world, it can be an instrument by which people themselves identify not only their needs but their potential for participation in their community. It can also operate as a means by which different organisations can work together in a more collaborative way to identify needs which, if met, may improve the circumstances of a large number of people.

In the current move towards community-based health care and collective views of health there are a number of challenges for all organisations that work with people. These challenges include the need to develop shared vision about the end point of their endeavours. With this shared vision, they can ultimately identify the means by which they will reach this goal. In order to do this they must be clear about the perspectives that underpin their work so that those who read the results of their endeavours can make informed judgements about the validity of the findings. Organisations must work together with each other and with the people whom they serve with no single organisation or group claiming the 'moral high ground'. This may prove difficult for medicine (and indeed nursing) but is a key feature of work for public health. This chapter will explore these issues in relation to assessing health needs by exploring the concepts that underpin health needs assessment to demonstrate the gap that can exist within and between disciplines, agencies and organisations when assumed to be working on the same endeavour. The chapter will then highlight and discuss the need for partnership of people within the assessment of their own needs before identifying some potentially participatory models of assessment. In conclusion, the chapter will examine the drive for collaborative working and its potential for enriching the assessment of communities' health needs.

Conceptual Dilemmas

Health needs assessment has been described as both complex and multidimensional. The complexity stems from the different methods of data collection that are employed as well as the notion that the resulting assessment is dependent upon who performs the health needs assessment and why. Perhaps most importantly the complexity arises from the lack of universal meaning of both 'health' and 'needs'.

It is considered multidimensional because needs can be identified at various levels, that is individual, family, group, community and wider populations. A further dimension is that the approach may be 'top-down' where the process is driven by health and social care professionals or 'bottom-up' where the process is led by individuals, family, groups, community and wider populations themselves. Other dimensions can be identified within the purposes for which health needs assessment is and can be used.

Health

There is a plethora of theories about the nature of health, some underpinned by a bio-medical approach (variations on the theme of absence of disease) and others underpinned by a humanist approach (variations on the theme of personal achievement of potential). Generally theories about health can be divided into two major areas. There are those which view health as the result of individual endeavours in terms of maintaining health by 'doing the right thing' as advised by perhaps medical practitioners and other health protagonists. The alternative viewpoint is the social health model which recognises that the many structures which exist in a complex society have an impact not only on people's well-being but also on their potential to support their own health. Clearly in health needs assessment what you find will be dependent upon what you look for.

The prevailing view of health may be impacted upon by various experiences, beliefs and values, all of which may be influenced by a powerful media, government policies and the 'spin' that accompanies them as well as the way that powerful groups interpret history and what may be learned from it. Some argue that 'health' as a notion is becoming so all-encompassing that it is losing any real meaning (Seedhouse, 1997) whereas others would view it as the cumulative result of the way that we view life and the experience that it offers (fairly all-encompassing!) (Antonovsky, 1987, 1993) and that the pathogenic approach is too narrow a view.

As an example of how concepts can drive policy and ultimately service delivery and indeed common parlance and culture, we need look no further than the NHS and Community Care Act (DoH, 1990). Harrison (1996) takes the optimistic view that the supposed shift from service-driven to needs-led patterns in the delivery of care was to address three basic problems. Specifically these problems were: professional dominance over resource allocation, lack of motivation for efficiency gains and a failure to provide choice for the users of services. However, this legislation, under the guise of tailoring services to need, successfully managed to separate people's social circumstances from their health status. This led to an immense amount of costly time spent trying to discern 'health needs' from 'social needs'. This cost may have been deemed to be worthwhile to the government of the time because the division of need in this way meant the saving of large amounts of money. The meeting of health needs, would remain 'free at the point of delivery', from 'cradle to grave' but people could not of course expect the same for simple social needs. This paved the way for the culture change which was to come in which people would be expected to contribute financially to their own care and some chronically disabled people were discharged from hospital care into nursing home care because their needs were considered to be 'social'. Certainly a more honest approach to this policy may have been achieved if concepts had been clarified at the outset. However, that may have not achieved the desired result for the government at the time.

Need

Bradshaw's (1972) taxonomy of need, from a sociological viewpoint is generally considered relevant to both those who deliver care and those who use it. He distinguishes between four different types of need:

1   *Normative needs* are those defined by experts or professionals in relation to an agreed standard. Individuals or groups falling below these agreed standards are said to be 'in need'.

2   *Felt needs* are those identified by individuals themselves. These needs may or may not be expressed in action.

3   *Expressed needs* are those felt needs which have been acted upon by individuals or groups.

4   *Comparative needs* are those of a particular group of individuals relative to those of another group with similar characteristics.

Bradshaw (1994) continues that when people use the term 'need' they mean a combination of each of these four definitions and that in practice real need exists when each of these four elements are present at the same time. Criticisms made of Bradshaw's typology are the difficulty of forming clear comparable criteria for needs assessment (Billings and Cowley, 1995) and the lack of methodological evidence to suggest the concepts could be operationalised in a meaningful way (Thayer, 1973). However, what this

typology does help us to understand is that there is more than one perspective on what is 'needed' by any individual, group or community and
in order to gain a full picture of need, all perspectives should be part of the
equation.

Braye and Preston-Shoot (1995) however suggest that where service
users needs remain within the judgement of professionals any needs
assessment is destined to be inadequate. They identify how, even when
'participation' is encouraged, users do not control the process and their
wishes are rarely determinative either in defining need or how it will be
met. Many areas of need, particularly where need is focused on individual
rather than collective experience, are likely to exclude, for example, the cultural pressures which have disabling effects on women, disabled people
and minority groups. Emotional needs may be considered irrelevant, and
expressed and felt needs may be viewed as 'wishes' and therefore considered of less value. This professional domination is suggested by Braye and
Preston-Shoot (1995) to have the iatrogenic effect of leaving people feeling
isolated, blamed and misunderstood.

Clarke (1998) goes further and highlights the notion of 'professional
blindness' in terms of the level of professional intervention in areas of
social need. They argue that professionals are simply using a medical
model of dependence under a different guise. This dispossesses the poor
communities of their role in articulating their social concerns and has led
to the consolidation of the power of professionals, the glorification of professional expertise and the inhibition of social innovation. In other words,
the professionals are colluding at maintaining people in their poverty and
offering only stability to the status quo rather than real social change
which will improve people's lives.

Assessment

Assessment in itself is a complex issue that is inclined to be profession specific. Doctors may talk about scientific methods and the diagnostic process,
while nurses use the term assessment to include gathering information
(data) from clients/patients and carers through observation, interviewing
and listening to cues (Ross and Mackenzie, 1996). Indeed, any profession
will bring to the notion of assessment its own value and belief system.

Assessment at an individual level is entirely different to assessment at a
community level and will render completely different data. However,
assessment at a community level is also highly politically charged. Health
needs assessment is the premise on which many services are being determined but we cannot claim to have a foolproof and inclusive way of
assessing health needs. It is more likely within this kind of approach that

assessment of health need will meet the requirements of the majority and that there will be groups of people who are excluded from the whole machinery of assessment either because of their invisibility or because of their lack of participation in the mainstream processes.

We may be in danger of substituting one form of service-driven provision with another. Health Action Zones, Education Action Zones, Sure Start, and many of the other innovations and projects which are currently vaunted to be meeting needs, are all underpinned by some form of assessment which must be submitted to justify the financing of the project. These assessments, in order to secure the funding, must demonstrate a need for the particular 'service' that is being bid for which means that the assessment is in danger of being skewed towards the particular service. This may be resolved by the short-term nature of the projects in that assessment should be ongoing and where the needs change, so will the service. However, what is likely to happen is that where the money is about to come to an end, an assessment may be submitted which secures the funding but does not necessarily truly identify the need. If professionals control the assessment, the assessment will surely continue to demonstrate the need for professional intervention.

Participatory Approaches to Health Needs Assessment

The drive for people to at best control but at least participate in identifying their own needs is clear. Participatory models might be argued to be somewhat less about resource allocation than other models and more about an open approach and a different way of looking at possible need and then creatively working with populations on how that need might be met. However, while participation has to be demonstrated in order to successfully gain funding for projects and initiatives, most participatory approaches are local and small scale and arguably people may find it difficult to discern the results of their participation.

Most researchers advocate the use of multiple data collection methods, that is qualitative and quantitative, in order for each to compensate for the others shortcomings (Leininger, 1985). The danger of course is that the qualitative (which is almost by definition the smaller scale) research, will be subsumed among the large scale epidemiological or socio-economic approaches which use large populations giving what may seem a greater weight of evidence and, of course, because of the way that they are collected and collated offer that evidence in favour of a medical professional interventionist approach.

Focus Groups

Focus groups may be one way of involving local people in health needs assessment and have the potential for gaining a wider range of information and experience. As a form of qualitative research, focus groups are essentially group interviews involving 5 to 15 people, debating topics that are supplied by the facilitator, that is the researcher (Thomas, 1993; Polit and Hungler, 1995). The facilitator's role is to introduce the topics for discussion and facilitate the contributions of the participants. The fundamental data produced by focus groups are transcripts of the group discussions (Morgan, 1991).

Focus groups are widely used in health research to study a whole range of health issues with groups of all ages, ethnicity and varying demographic conformations. Focus groups are considered a useful method because they provide a practical way to study people's knowledge, opinions, constructs, ideas, feelings and motives about health as well as their actions, as expressed in their own words. However, Jordan *et al.* (1998) argue that for the most part focus groups encourage discussion of uninformed opinion.

The perennial problem with any participative research and particularly with focus groups is the danger of hearing only the people who are most able to register their demands or needs at the expense of the less articulate. Within focus groups, it would need confidence and an expert facilitator to ensure that even with the small group, the quieter members were able to express their opinion and experiences if they came into conflict with others who were more assertive. Similarly there is an issue of how access to the group was gained and the problem of how to ensure that there is at least some safeguard of only eliciting the opinions of community (often self-styled) 'leaders'.

Rapid Participatory appraisal

Rapid participatory appraisal is a qualitative technique for community assessment (Bowling, 1997b) and has been used to establish the foundation for an ongoing relationship between service purchasers, providers and the public (Picken and St Ledger, 1993). The aims of rapid participatory appraisal include, gaining an insight into the community's own perspective on its priority needs and translating these findings into action. It is also possible, according to Murray *et al.* (1994), for this method to establish a continuing relationship between those commissioning services, professionals delivering the service and local communities.

The key features of rapid participatory appraisal are that they involve interviews with key informants, use focus groups and observation of the area to build up the profile and requires involvement of the practice team.

This method involves collecting information on nine areas of activity in four 'layers' (Figure 7.1). The bottom layer defines the composition of the community, how it is organised and its capacities to act. The second layer covers the sociological factors that influence health and embraces the notion that social and environmental factors influence the general health and well-being of a community. The third layer encompasses data on the existence, coverage, accessibility and acceptability of services. These allow evaluation of the effectiveness of present provision and provide a method of assessing what could usefully be changed. The top layer is concerned with national, regional and local policies which change periodically. Hence, these influences are dependent on what is happening at the time. The pyramid shape serves as a reminder that the success of this process depends on the building of planning procedures that are based on a foundation of strong community information (Gillam and Murray, 1996).

In common with other participatory approaches rapid appraisal is small scale and located within deprived areas. One of the weaknesses identified by Murray *et al.* (1994) is the time that it takes and the commitment required from team members. Additionally it is possible, as Jordan *et al.* (1998) point out, for organisers to have undue influence over the outcomes of this kind of exercise, simply in the nature of the questions that they ask and how they ask them. Jordan *et al.* (1998) also raise an important issue

Figure 7.1   Rapid participatory assessment pyramid (Murray *et al.*, 1994)

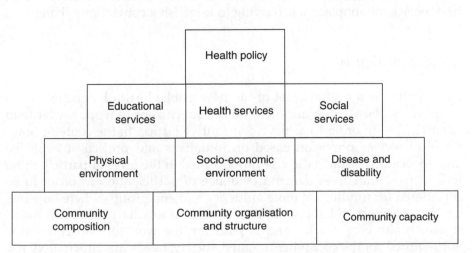

with regard to all participatory approaches and that is the absence of relevant training. They identify that working with groups representing different community interests demands considerable skills and flexibility, and health professionals (who are most commonly the professionals undertaking this kind of exercise) are poorly prepared for this.

Citizen's Juries

There are several difficulties with the above methods. Not least of these is that the approaches do not identify the necessity, or at least the desirability for choices and decisions to be informed in any way. One of the issues that is recognised to impact on people's abilities to make decisions and choices and even to participate fully in society is lack of information, yet many of the participatory models simply ask for people's uninformed opinions. People, particularly disadvantaged groups, do not have access to unfettered information which would help them to make informed decisions. There are hard choices to be made within any service or community which involves social and ethical dilemmas, and the public have the right to the information that may impact on those choices. Leneghan *et al.* (1996) suggest that citizen's juries are a way of overcoming some of these problems. Citizen's juries and similar panels of members of the public place respondents in the situation where they are informed about the issues and choices at stake. They must then deliberate with others to arrive at a recommendation. This method is an attempt to collect the views of the public not necessarily as they are, but as they might be if information and the opportunity for discussion were available. Citizen's juries should not be mistaken for some of the manipulative 'consultation exercises' which have been commonplace when trying to establish a contentious change.

Illusion of Equity

Participation is a central tenet of the new public health language and in many ways places a responsibility on certain citizens to work harder than other citizens in order to achieve distributive justice. In the contemporary mode of service provision based on initiatives and projects it could be argued that provision is directly proportional to the level of participation. Indeed most initiatives demand evidence of participation in order to be considered for funding. In more affluent areas and groups where housing, leisure, transport and social support as well as auxiliary and even mainstream health care can be, and is paid for, the work of participation is not required. In the consumer-oriented society, needs are anticipated and provided for by commercial groups who have a vested interest in ensuring provision fits the need. The language and the culture of power and control is the language of the already privileged. Most marginalised groups are not used to being asked for their opinion and simple one off consultation is unlikely to have a major impact either at the level of process or outcome. Indeed they may have a deleterious effect on longer term effectiveness when local people do not recognise any result for their efforts in participation, partly because the results are subsumed but also because workers who undertake the assessment do not have direct control over resources.

Almost more important than methods is the notion of sustainability in local participation. Structures should be in place at a national and local democratic level which work constantly to inform and enable participation. There is a level of disenfranchisement in Britain among certain groups which will take a great deal of work and building of trust to overcome but if we are to truly hope for participation in societal structures then this is where it should start. Participation is not something that should be left to local individual professionals in trying to elicit the opinions of uninformed citizens who may have lost trust in a system which clearly devalues them in every other way.

Collaboration

In order to work with communities effectively, professionals must use frameworks to understand and secure inter-professional and inter-agency working to share data for a richer understanding of the needs of communities. The fragmentation that exists in professional data collecting does a disservice to communities.

The emphasis on collaborative working in recent years (DoH, 1999a; NHSE, 1999) now challenges the previous and divisive paradigm of 'tribalism' among the health professionals and statutory agencies (Beattie, 1991). Contemporary government policy demands collaborative working on areas of identified health and health care needs in local areas through the joint Local Health Authority and Primary Care Group/Trusts HImPs (DoH, 1999b). This necessitates a unified and broad concept of both health and health care need assessment so that multi-agency groups may work together towards promoting the health of the population as a whole. Furthermore, there is increasing emphasis directed towards targeting inequalities in health and health care (DoH, 1999a). Hence, the assessment of health and health care need from a health practitioner's perspective may arise at three levels – individual, family or group, community or wider population.

Similar to participation, collaboration is a requirement of many bids for funding for public health projects. However it is at the level of the individual that collaboration has perhaps been forced on to the agenda in the nature of single assessment of health needs of, for example, the older person and children in need, where social services, health services and other vested interests are expected to work together in producing a cohesive assessment of need.

Braye and Preston-Shoot (1995) identify some key issues for collaboration which can be used either at a single assessment (individual) level or group or community level. The key concepts that they advocate are unsurprisingly similar to the issues for community participation. They generally can be distilled into a development of shared vision, a commitment to power sharing, partnership, and prevention of maintaining only one world view as well as transparent decision making systems and distinction between task and process bearing in mind that the work can be of advantage to both.

It is unrealistic to expect communities to work with professionals if professionals are unable to emulate the models of co-operation by working together. It would be simple to identify the structural barriers to this kind of collaboration, that is lack of shared budgets, mistrust of different organisations, litigation culture. However, there are also barriers at the individual staff level where simple communication with each other, professional updating and information seeking, willingness to make decisions and lobbying of their own organisation would make the straightforward difference at the grass roots level. This is something for which individual practitioners can take responsibility and surely asking practitioners to take the same kind of responsibility as we ask disadvantaged communities to do is not asking too much.

Conclusion

Health needs assessment is a popular and complex concept which is often undertaken with an assumption of agreement between the people involved. There appears to be a dominant 'world view' of health and its determinants and this chapter claims that it is this powerful view that underpins what in reality is health *care* needs assessment in Britain today. This approach to assessment is about identification of services and rationing those services according to perceived need. Health needs assessment on the other hand is about identifying need as perceived by people themselves, exploring how this impacts on their lives and developing creative solutions to the problems and difficulties identified.

The process is politically charged both in its antecedents and in its processes. It arose out of the need to more effectively target provision but as a result of various social changes and pressures has evolved into a more democratic principle. The democratic principle is not yet however underpinned by robust methods. Epidemiological and socio-economic methods prevail as the most powerful in terms of resource allocation. Other more participatory methods are developing but are as yet at a rudimentary stage in their ability to achieve what they set out to achieve.

It is recognised that in areas where multi-agencies are involved, cautious handling as to the varying interpretations and approaches to 'need' are required for effective inter-sectoral collaboration and appropriate provision of services for users (Lightfoot, 1995). This calls for joint training in some areas so that varying professionals can understand each other's work and that each holds a common, focused joint strategy for the improvement of health and reduction of inequality. Community consultation is paramount in defining those issues that affect their lives and in establishing appropriate services, which are socially and culturally acceptable. This assists in redressing inequalities in both the quality and access to health care services and combine action on the social determinants that impact on the health of individuals and communities.

References

Antonovsky, A. (1993) The Structure and Properties of the Sense of Coherence Scale. *Social Science and Medicine*, 36, 6, 725–33.

Antonovsky, A. (1987) The Salutogenic Perspective: Toward a New View of Health and Illness. *Advances*, 4, 1, 47–55.

Beattie, A. (1991) Knowledge and Control in Health Promotion: A Test Case for Social Policy and Social Theory. In Gabe, J., Calnan, M. and Bury, M. (eds) *The Sociology of the Health Service*. London: Routledge.

Billings, J. (1996) *Profiling for Health: the Process and Practice*. London: Health Visitors Association.

Billings, J.R. and Cowley, S. (1995) Approaches to Community Needs Assessment: a Literature Review. *Journal of Advanced Nursing*, 22, 721–30.

Bowling, A. (1997a) *Research Methods in Health. Investigating Health and Health Services*. Buckingham: Open University Press.

Bowling, A. (1997b) *Measuring Health. A Review of Life Measurement Scales* (2nd edn). Buckingham and Philadelphia: Open University Press.

Bradshaw, J. (1972) A taxonomy of Social Need. In McLachlan, G. (ed.) *Problems and Progress in Medical Care*. Oxford: Nuffield Provincial Hospital Trust.

Bradshaw, J. (1994). The Conceptualisation and Measurement of Need: A Social Policy Perspective. In Popay, J. and Williams, G. (eds) *Researching the People's Health*. London: Routledge.

Braye, S. and Preston-Shoot, M. (1995) *Empowering Practice in Social Care*. Buckingham: Open University Press.

Clarke, S. (1998) Community Development and Health Professionals. In Symonds, A. and Kelly, A. (eds) *The Social Construction of Community Care*. Basingstoke: Macmillan – now Palgrave.

DoH (Department of Health) (1990) *Caring for People: Implementation Document – Assessment and Case Management*. London: HMSO.

DoH (Department of Health) (1997) *The New NHS: Modern. Dependable*. London: The Stationery Office.

DoH (Department of Health) (1999a) *Saving Lives: Our Healthier Nation*. London: The Stationery Office.

DoH (Department of Health) (1999b) *Making a Difference. Strengthening the Nursing, Midwifery and Health Visiting Contribution to Health and Health Care*. London: The Stationery Office.

DoH (Department of Health) (2001) *The Report of the Chief Medical Officer's Project to Strengthen the Public Health Function*. London: The Stationery Office.

Gillam, S.J. and Murray, S.A. (1996) *Needs Assessment in General Practice*. London: Royal College of General Practitioners (Occasional Paper 73).

Harrison, L. (1996) Needs Assessment and the NHS: Context and Change. In Burton, P. and Harrison, L. (eds) (1996) *Identifying Health Needs. New Community Based Approaches*. York: The Policy Press.

Jordan, J., Dowswell, T., Harrison, S., Lilford, R.J. and Mort, M. (1998) Whose priorities? Listening to Users and the Public. *British Medical Journal*, 316, 1668–1670.

Leininger, M.M. (1985) *Qualitative Research Methods in Nursing*. New York: Grune and Stratton.

Leneghan, J., New, B. and Mitchell, E. (1996) Setting Priorities: Is There a Role for Citizens' Juries? *British Medical Journal*, 312, 1591–93.

Lightfoot, J. (1995) Identifying Needs and Setting Priorities: Issues of Theory, Policy and Practice. *Health and Social Care*, 3, 105–14.

Marti-Costa, S. and Serrano-Garcia, I. (1995) Needs Assessment and Community Development: An Ideological Perspective. In Rothman, J., Erlich, J.L. and Tropman, J.E. (eds) (1995) *Strategies of Community Intervention* (5th edn). Illinois: Peacock Publishers.

Morgan, M. (1991) Sociological Investigations. In Holland, W.W., Deletes, R. and Knox, G. (eds) *The Oxford Textbook of Public Health* (2nd edn) (1991) *Vol. 2. Methods of Public Health*, Oxford: Oxford University Press.

Murray, S.A., Tapson, J., Turnbull, L., McCallum, J. and Little, A. (1994). Listening to Local Voices: Adapting Rapid Appraisal to Assess Health and Social Needs in General Practice. *British Medical Journal*, 308, 698–700.

NHSE (1999) *Making a Difference*. London: NHSE.

NHSME (NHS Management Executive) (1992) *Local Voices: The Views of Local People in the Purchasing for Health*. London: NHSME.

Picken, C. and St Ledger, S. (1993). *Assessing Health Need Using the Lifecycle Framework*. Oxford: Oxford University Press.

Polit, D.F. and Hungler, B.P. (1995) *Essentials of Nursing Research. Methods, Appraisal and Utilisation*. Philadelphia: Lippincott.

Ross, F. and Mackenzie, A. (1996) *Nursing in Primary Health Care. Policy into Practice*. London and New York: Routledge.

Seedhouse, D. (1997) *Health Promotion. Philosophy, Prejudice and Practice*. Chichester: Wiley.

Stevens, A. and Gabbay, J. (1991) Needs Assessment Needs Assessment. *Health Trends*, 23, 1, 20–3.

Thayer, R. (1973) Measuring Need in Social Services. *Social and Economic Administration*, 7 May, 91–105.

Thomas, J. (1993) *Doing Critical Ethnography*. Newbury Park, California: Sage Publications.

8

Social Exclusion and Public Health

JOHN COSTELLO

The key points discussed in this chapter are:

- the origins of social exclusion and a description of the processes involved

- the major reasons underpinning social exclusion and the links between social exclusion and public health

- the contrasting characteristics of social exclusion and an identification of those members of society who are socially excluded.

Introduction

Writers have variously described public health as a new morality whereby they are capable of participating actively in the social life of their society (Peterson and Lupton, 1996). Others argue that health is a response of people to their environment (Milio, 1986) and a process which includes a series of transitions between productive health and state of complete well-being (Beaglehole and Bonita, 1997). Richman in Chapter 1 identified that public health involved communities, societies and countries striving to create an environment whereby optimum health conditions can be sustained within the resources available. Essentially (as the preceding chapters of this book have highlighted) in a broad sense, public health may be seen as a series of processes in which socio-political forces strive to attain the best effective strategies for ensuring individual and community health. These processes incorporate physical, mental, spiritual, and social well-being and in doing so embrace what many refer to as a holistic approach, although critics of public health strategies would argue that, for many, public health scientists are primarily orientated towards physical disease. Public health in its widest context, however, is more than the treatment of physical disease. It is concerned with prevention, education, promotion and eradication of the social issues underpinning the enduring health problems closely associated with disease causation such as poverty and all forms of social exclusion.

The purpose of this chapter is to examine social exclusion as a contemporary phenomenon, tracing its origins and attempting to elicit why people are socially excluded as well as identifying the links between social exclusion and public health. The chapter examines the characteristics of social exclusion and asks a number of questions, such as who are socially excluded and what is the Government doing about this major social problem? In attempting to answer these questions I consider patterns of social exclusion using three authentic case studies of people who, by government definition, are socially excluded. The case studies enable a more practical and focused view to be made of the differing ways in which people become socially excluded, but also the reader is able to see the common elements of each. The chapter examines poverty and unemployment which, when the reader considers the issues raised by the case studies, play an integral part in perpetuating social exclusion.

The latter part of the chapter looks critically at the response made by the Labour Government in setting up Social Exclusion Units (SEUs). The argument advanced is that the function of SEUs in monitoring the experiences of the socially disaffected and gathering data on the so-called socially excluded draws attention to the outcomes of exclusion without dealing with the more complex social conditions. In critically analysing this political approach to the perceived problem of social exclusion, I contend that it is not resolved by the creation of an outcome-driven government think tank. Ultimately, the issue of social exclusion may be seen as a by-product of an advanced capitalist society concerned more with self-determination and less with critically analysing the root causes of social exclusion. By creating SEUs, the government is seen to be taking action based on identifying the needs of the excluded, but not addressing the issues giving rise to social exclusion, thus failing to address the real issue of developing routes towards social inclusion. This creates the illusion that people rather than the social system are the problem. The emphasis is placed on 'doing something' and not on creating space for needy people, who are seen as 'the problem' not the lack of resources available to accommodate them and assimilate their needs within wider society. Here, we see links with the problem of vulnerability and the needs of the homeless and the disenfranchised, such as, members of ethnic minorities (see Costello *et al*. Chapter 4).

Broadly speaking, social exclusion may be seen as the lack or denial of access to the kinds of social relations, social customs and activities that the majority of people within a given society enjoy. Since at least the 1980s,

Britain has developed a worldwide reputation for being a socially divided country, reflecting many of the characteristics of social exclusion. Internationally, with the exception of New Zealand, the pace of social and economic inequality in Britain is faster than any industrialised country. Over the period, 1979 to 1992, the poorest 20–30 per cent of the population failed to benefit from economic growth, in contrast with the rest of the post-war period (Joseph Rowntree Foundation, 1995). What we see today is an 'inverse need' relationship. Those in greatest need of social welfare reform receive the least. Vulnerable members of society have their needs managerially dealt with by government strategies (social exclusion categorisation), missing out the need to resolve the underlying social issues that gave rise to their vulnerability in the first place.

Social Exclusion and Public Health

The health of any nation can be measured in terms of both mortality and morbidity, which include the experiences of more vulnerable members of society (see Spanswick's chapter). Spanswick draws attention to the problems faced by those who experience ever-increasing deprivation, and physical and mental ill health. Governments and their agents, through analysis of epidemiological data, constantly monitor mortality, morbidity and the health of communities, families and individuals. By examining disease causation and its spread in this way, public health workers are able to control and monitor illness. Much of this data is disease focused and little account is taken of underlying social problems such as poverty, poor housing and social class differences which influence illness causation (Peterson and Lupton, 1996; Benyon, 1999).

The historical evidence almost overwhelmingly suggests that socio-economic factors play a major role in health. The majority of diseases, which caused death in the nineteenth century, were as a result of urban poverty and the filthy conditions of the working class poor who populated small areas of industrialised cities living in overcrowded conditions and squalid environments, typical of present-day Asian and Far Eastern 'sweat shop' countries such as Indonesia and Korea. Workers in nineteenth-century England lived, as many Asian workers do today, in conditions which perpetuate disease exacerbated by long working hours, poor nutrition and constant stress. Contrasting this scenario to the present day, we see the victims of poverty and unemployment are stigmatised and the creation of what Giddens (1997) calls 'the underclass'. This gives tacit permission for certain sections of society, notably the tabloid press, to blame these people for their own ills creating the situation of a modern-day workhouse.

One of the most significant reports on health inequalities, which also highlights the plight of people who may be considered socially excluded, was the Acheson Report (Acheson, 1988) (the *Independent Inquiry into Inequalities in Health*). This report pointed the way to understanding the nature of social inequalities in Britain, arguing that the origins of health inequalities stem from individual life-styles, community networks and the socio-economic and environmental conditions that perpetuate the lack of social mobility of certain disadvantaged groups. These, as Haggart and Richman point out in their chapters, are key public health issues. The Acheson Report focuses on the interrelationships between these three areas that largely help to identify ways in which individuals and groups become socially excluded. Poor standards of living, particularly for young families in deprived areas that become susceptible to downward spiralling are often caused or made worse by prevailing negative economic conditions. This combined with life-style factors such as a reliance on drugs, poor eating habits and chronic illness, militate towards a negative pattern of social action which can be reversed if sufficient help and attention is paid to the causes and processes which push certain individuals and social groups towards social exclusion.

What is Social Exclusion?

Social exclusion is a term used to identify individuals and social groups whose life and health care experiences are influenced by a range of social welfare issues such as poverty, unemployment and social deprivation. People seen as being socially excluded often share similar life experiences. These recurring features of the socially excluded have been shown to include a lack of employment and social skills, low income, tendency to crime, poor health and family breakdown. In broad terms, Mason *et al.* (2001) contend that social exclusion involves individuals and groups in society who, despite being part of mainstream society, become marginalised and disaffected from the prevailing culture, whereas the SEU define it as: 'A shorthand term for what can happen when people or areas suffer from a combination of linked problems such as unemployment, poor skills, low incomes, poor housing high crime, bad health and family breakdown' (SEU, 2001).

Definitions and explanations obviously vary according to the social and political perspective taken by those making the definition. However, there are often commonalities in definitions which make it useful for the reader to identify the key issues associated with social exclusion despite the political connotations.

In both definitions, social exclusion involves people who played an active part in society but, for a number of reasons such as living in poverty for many years as a result of low income or unemployment, find themselves at crisis point. These crisis points can arise from marital breakdown, family dysfunction or sudden unemployment necessitating a change of circumstances such as homelessness. These place the individual at odds with the rest of society. (The following case studies depict a number of such scenarios and circumstances.) When individual circumstances are examined carefully, that is, how and why the person became homeless, unemployed or destitute, it becomes easier to identify how to tackle and thus prevent further exclusion but only if there is a degree of understanding of the real underlying issues involved.

What Does Social Exclusion Involve?

The SEU's definition reflects a number of interesting features of government thinking. First, it does not include all forms of social exclusion. Second, it may be argued that in defining key areas such as health, crime, unemployment and skills, the Government is making the link between these social problems, although perhaps not recognising some of the complexities underpinning the causation of each. An illustration of this is the use of illegal drugs by people from a range of social backgrounds, together with the reasons why people tend to use drugs that may not in any way be due to poverty. It is, however, interesting to consider the political experiences in order to collectively identify a range of social ills and make a public commitment to tackling them. This allows government not only to be seen to be challenging social problems but also to enable them to claim that any future falls in incidence can be attributed to the initial assumption that all forms of social deviance emanate from and are perhaps closely associated with, social exclusion. Finally, as this chapter will identify, it is important to recognise that the problems initially linked to social exclusion change over time, although often it is not always easy to become reintegrated back into society once the process of (socially excluded) labelling has occurred. It is also necessary to examine interrelationships between each of the areas of social division highlighting both their uniqueness and interrelated nature. The SEU Report (2001) points out that: 'The most important characteristic of social exclusion is that these problems are linked and mutually reinforcing, and can combine to create a complex and fast moving vicious circle. Only when this process is properly understood and addressed will policies really be effective'.

In its 1999 review of progress (SEU, 1999a) the government rhetoric produced an all-embracing image suggesting that the relationship between poverty and other social deprivations was well established. Clearly the implications of low income mean that the poor are not able to share the same resources and opportunities as others, such as home ownership, high educational attainment and secure employment. The review of progress, while acknowledging these issues, failed to highlight the 'stand-alone' properties of these social deprivations.

Who Are the Socially Excluded?

The interlinked factors of social exclusion go wider than an identification of the types of people and the social groups at risk. One of the problems in developing the latter approach is that social problems such as unemployment may be prescribed for certain types of individuals, such as those who underachieve at education and the job market, together with those with limited access to services. People who are socially excluded share certain social characteristics such as ill health and stress which may be seen as the human cost of social exclusion. Table 8.1 identifies individuals/ social groups who experience social exclusion.

The list of the socially excluded needs to be interpreted more as a matrix and less in terms of comprehensiveness. Gregg and Wadsworth (1994) point out that those who grow up in low income families tend to become unemployed and also spend time in prison. Equally, evidence suggests that children from so-called broken homes or homes where there is recurrent conflict, such as an alcoholic family member, are more likely to offend, use drugs or become homeless (SEU, 2000). In this sense, it may be argued that for some people, in order to adapt and survive their circumstances, it becomes necessary to disengage from society. In doing so, it appears that such individuals have taken a conscious decision to drop out

Table 8.1   Individuals/social groups who experience social
exclusion

- People who grow up in low income families and become unemployed
- Individuals who experience family conflict
- Lone parents
- Young people in care
- Children experiencing problems at school, particularly those excluded
- Ex-prisoners
- People from ethnic minorities
- People with mental health issues
- Older people
- Disabled people
- People living in urban and rural areas

of society when, in actuality, society has disenfranchised and rejected such people who, after living on the margins, find themselves unable to continue and sustain their existence.

What Are Social Exclusion Units?

The Labour Government announced in August 1997 that it intended to set up a unit to tackle social exclusion in Britain. The SEU was set up in December that year and consisted of 12 full-time and four part-time civil servants and people outside of government; all of whom had front-line experience of dealing with social exclusion problems. The aim of the SEU was to focus attention on individuals and social groups whom it was felt experienced social exclusion. Initially, a number of priorities were identified including truants who became excluded from school, those living in deprived housing estates throughout the country and rough sleepers.

Under the auspices of the Prime Minister, Tony Blair, who played a major part in setting up the SEU, it was made clear to the public that this unit would specifically tackle the wide-ranging issues emanating from social divisions within British society, specifically poverty and low income, which have the effect of marginalising individuals, families and the community to the point where they are perceived to be socially excluded from mainstream society. The background to the SEU was based on the need of a New Labour Government who came into office determined to tackle the deepening social crisis caused by wide-ranging social inequalities; notably, income inequality, poverty and increased drug abuse, together with a range of social issues which impacted on personal and community health. In the mid 1990s comparisons with European neighbours in relation to social and health inequalities showed that Britain had the worst record for children growing up in jobless households, teenage pregnancy and drug use among young people, together with one of the highest rates of adult illiteracy (SEU, 1999b), increasing child poverty and record numbers of people sleeping rough. These accumulated social problems not only constitute considerable social suffering but also have major public financial implications. The remit of the SEU was to develop and improve government responses towards the socially excluded. The priority areas were school truancy, rough sleepers, poor neighbourhoods, teenage pregnancy and unemployed 16 to 18 year olds not in education or training schemes.

One of the key aims of the SEU is to promote and evaluate research evidence likely to bring about a change in the social trends which perpetuate social exclusion. The review of SEUs in 1999 drew attention to the progress made in tackling social exclusion. The unit initiated 18 policy action teams

(PATs) to specifically monitor and co-ordinate activity on sleeping rough and teenage pregnancy, emphasising the need to focus on young people (SEU, 2000). A wealth of information, together with these reports, is available to policy makers in social welfare and health care professionals by way of keeping abreast of the SEUs work.

Understanding Patterns of Social Exclusion: A Case Study Approach

One way of identifying linkages in the way that individuals encounter social problems and become socially excluded is by using authentic case study scenarios which, as Yin (1994) argues, enables insights into the social experiences of individuals/social groups to be made, examining their social world in order to develop a more realistic perspective.

To enable me to reproduce authentic case study scenarios, I contacted a number of informants via people who were both known to me and willing to help in approaching individuals willing to be interviewed about their experiences. I used these contacts at Nacro and the *Big Issue* in the north as 'go-betweens' to introduce willing informants to me. The third party obtained informed consent from the participants and I verified their willingness to participate when we first met. (This type of approach is described in more detail in Costello and Horne, 2001.) In some cases, when attempting to answer research questions with what Moore and Miller (1999) call doubly vulnerable populations (those who experience more than one factor that diminishes their autonomy) the need arises to ask members of the research population themselves.

I chose to focus on three informants: One (Ken) was an ex-prisoner who, as a recidivist, had a long experience of prison life and agreed to become an informant partly because he felt he wanted to share his experiences but also because he wanted to impress his probation officer who was the go-between I had to contact. The second was a young man of 16, Stephen, who had spent time in care and was currently in short-term foster care. The third, Stan, I met while he was selling the *Big Issue*. He agreed to be interviewed when I invited him to lunch, accepted my offer on the basis that there is no such thing as a free lunch, but I had to buy a copy of the *Big Issue*!

Ken

Ken was a 51-year-old who had been in prison on a number of occasions, mainly for burglary and petty theft. Ken looked much older than his age, was pale and had a very harsh, unproductive cough. His criminal career began at 13 when he was caught shoplifting. He spent time in Borstal and had eight subsequent episodes in prison. Ken left school at 14 with no qualifications; he was a very poor reader although he had learnt to write short letters with help from the prison educationalists. He described himself as a manual labourer with no specific skills. He smoked 30 cigarettes a day and suffered from chronic obstructive pulmonary disease. Ken was known locally as a receiver of stolen goods. He described his childhood as 'a bit of a pain at times' but on the whole was reasonably happy. His father was an alcoholic who rarely held down a full time job and died from liver cirrhosis when Ken was 17. His mother was hard working but, said Ken 'clapped out with stress'. As a child Ken frequently stole money from her purse and was, he pointed out a pathological liar. Despite this, Ken's mum supported him both in and out of prison. His one sister had learning difficulties and although he was fond of her the family was not what he would call close. Twice married, Ken was currently living with a partner and her two children from a previous marriage. Ken felt that the prison warders referred to him as 'an old lag'. He seemed to find a peculiar comfort from being in prison. 'On the inside you know where you stand nearly all the time, life is much more simple on the inside.'

Stephen

I met Stephen while he was in foster care. Both foster parents and social worker gave consent to conducting the interview, which was based on Stephen's life experiences of being in care. Stephen was one of four children. From an early age attendance at school was spasmodic, either staying at home, playing truant or being excluded, for various reasons, such as causing an affray in the classroom or refusing to do as he was told. In secondary school he had poor concentration and was a poor reader, despite being statemented and receiving help. He lacked social skills, was hyperactive and often became uncontrollable in class. Some teachers refused to teach him because of his disruptive behaviour which resulted in him being referred to an educational psychologist and home lessons. His mother worked as a machinist at home. His father was often unemployed and, when in work, spent long periods away; when in the house, he found it hard to cope with four children. Stephen's parents found it hard to manage the family, always being short of money, they frequently rowed. Stephen's mum having suffered a nervous breakdown, was currently taking anti-depressants.

Stephen could not recall any single event which led to him being taken into care, but, at the age of eight, recalls his father walking out and his mother spending long periods in her bedroom. During this time his aunty looked after him and his younger sister, aged six. His older brother joined the army, his older sister (aged 15) ran away from home. Stephen was taken into care when he was 11, spending six months in a children's home. He was subsequently fostered by several couples who found him a challenge, but he was never adopted and despite keeping in touch with his mother (his father left the family home when Stephen was 13 and never returned) she expressed no desire to have him at home. Stephen eventually left home, became unemployed, experimented with soft drugs and was arrested and charged with possession and supplying cannabis to younger children.

Stan

Stan is a 29-year-old *Big Issue* seller currently sleeping rough in Manchester. Stan recalls a happy childhood and describes himself as 'a bit of a tearaway'. He often skipped school, was a poor attender, and despite saying he enjoyed it when he was there, left at 16 with no qualifications. He had two younger sisters and describes the family as being close but 'we all went our separate ways just after I left school'. His parents separated and then divorced, his father went to live in London. His mother took his two sisters with her to Hull and he worked as a market labourer in Manchester staying with his aunt and uncle. Stan had a succession of jobs, mainly because he got bored and could not keep up the monotonous routine. He saw little of his family for several years. Stan refuses to move to Hull to be near his mother and sisters, but keeps in touch, visiting his mum now and again, although he has not kept in touch with his father.

Recently, he became involved in the Manchester club scene and worked behind bars in many clubs, where he established a reputation for hard work and reliability. He used soft drugs and drank moderately. 'I wouldn't touch the heavy gear, it does you in'. When his aunty died Stan's uncle left Manchester and sold the house. Stan moved into a shared house in Manchester but in terms of work, things did not work out because he felt he could not get on 'with groups of people'. Stan describes himself as 'a bit of a loner who likes to do his own thing and be his own boss'. He has not had any long-term relationships, thinking he is probably a bit shy when it comes to girls. After he lost his job (due to a 'bit of fiddling') short of money, Stan stayed in a number of squats in and around the city and eventually an organisation called Life Share found him unfurnished accommodation where he was able to live, although he became unable to get further work. Currently, he is hoping to save enough money before the weather gets too cold to get him to Dublin where he has friends who will put him up and provide him with bar work. He likes selling the *Big Issue* (but hates the rain). Currently he is happy in his flat, but he feels sure he will end up back on the streets.

Characteristics of Social Exclusion

Many key issues arise from the case studies that focus on the origins of social exclusion which are illustrated in Table 8.2. As the case studies highlight, there is considerable difficulty in defining social exclusion as a singular entity. Hence, perhaps, why the Government chose to include rough sleepers as a very visible group considered socially excluded. Rough

Table 8.2 Characteristics of social exclusion

Rough sleepers
- 30–50% suffer mental health problems
- Only 38% have any educational qualifications
- Up to 50% have a serious alcohol problem
- Up to 80% have drug problems

Young runaways (compared with those who do not run away)
- Three times more likely to be regular truants
- Twice as likely to have been excluded from school
- One-and-a-half times more likely to come from a workless household
- Five times more likely to have drug related problems
- Three times more likely to have been in trouble with the police

Prisoners
- 56% of prisoners are unemployed before sentencing
- 50% have poor reading skills, 80% have poor writing skills
- 67% have poor numeracy skills
- 38% will be homeless on release
- 47% are in debt at the time of sentence
- 66% admit to using drugs (other than alcohol) in the year before imprisonment

Young people (who have been in care) are more likely to:
- Leave school without qualifications
- Become unemployed
- Become teenage parents (two-and-a-half times the average risk)
- End up in prison (26% of prisoners have been in care as children, compared with 2% of the total population)
- End up homeless (between one-quarter and one-third of rough sleepers have been looked after by local authorities as children)

Source: SEU (2001).

sleepers may be seen as those who find themselves sleeping rough on the streets, but for some there is an option to sleep in a house or home which for varying reasons they are not able to do; this may be due to poor family relations, as in Stephen's case. There is also a clear case for arguing that money is a key issue along with the means to secure a steady source of income. Other factors which can be drawn out of the experiences of many socially excluded individuals are alcohol dependence in the family (perhaps a parent), physical/psychological abuse in the home, marital breakdown, loss of a job, house repossession or different socialisation.

According to the SEU, characteristics of social exclusion indicate that the most important feature of each identified group is that many of the problems associated are linked and mutually reinforcing. The case studies show that in all three cases educational attainment was a key issue, together with a lack of family integration. However, the identified characteristics combine to create a matrix of complex self-enhancing issues. Why was Stan a 'bit of a tearaway' and which factors resulted in Ken becoming a petty criminal at an early age? Clearly these issues could be looked at in terms of the nature/nurture debate. In Ken's case his social environment as a child was poor but his social deprivation was no worse than many others. Ken admitted that he was easily led and influenced heavily by others because, as he admits, 'I am weak when it comes to making decisions for myself'. Essentially, some would argue that a combination of factors caused him to become a criminal in much the same way that Stan preferred a degree of social isolation. Could it be that Stan was a rather shy individual and nobody ever got round to discovering that he found it difficult to relate to others and form long-term relationships? Identifying the precise issue is perhaps not as valuable as considering how the combined effects of his life-style work towards keeping people like Stan excluded. In doing so, it may help others experiencing similar problems. Consequently, until the underlying processes are clearly understood, it is difficult to develop effective policies to prevent individuals spiralling into social exclusion. Another consideration to be made, relating to the statistics on social exclusion, concern the accuracy of government figures. Media reports (*Guardian*, 2001) accuse the Government's Rough Sleeping Unit (RSU) of 'fixing' its twice-yearly count of the street population in order to meet its heavily advertised target. The Government pledged to reduce the number of rough sleepers by two-thirds although, according to media reports, homeless workers claim that the RSU have threatened rough sleepers with police action if they did not move off the streets and move into a hostel/shelter on the night the RSU carried out their winter count. The media report claims that the RSU put homeless people into bed-and-breakfast accommodation for several nights before the actual count. The Government's 'homeless Tsar' Louise Casey denied all allegations.

In summary, it may be argued that social exclusion originates in situations where the individual or group has a family history indicative of problems between generations, perhaps where parents have experienced difficulties in coping with family life (see Table 8.3). In particular parents with children who have special needs often point out that they need special skills and support to deal with the myriad problems associated with bringing up a family when the services are not made available.

Social Exclusion and Mental Health

The SEU data says little about people with serious mental illness and those with disabilities and learning difficulties. It does however identify that

Table 8.3 The origins of social exclusion

- Socially disadvantaged through poverty or hardship
- Demonstrating physical or mental health issues
- Experiencing a number of social factors likely to impede social mobility such as poor housing, unemployment, lack of education, life-style issues such as truancy or drug taking which are likely to perpetuate social exclusion
- Where there is evidence of family problems and difficulties in parent/child relations

socially excluded groups suffer from significantly higher levels of stress and mental health problems. Stress levels are rarely measured accurately, although it is not surprising that many people with mental health problems also experience social isolation and live in areas of deprivation with high crime levels, poor standards of housing and low public health resources. Evans and Repper (2000) suggest that some of the key issues focused on by the SEU such as poverty and unemployment are intricately linked with mental health. These authors cite the 1998 white paper *Modernizing Mental Health* and identify the link between the stigma of mental illness and the failure to understand its causes, pointing out that these issues can lead to further discrimination and social exclusion. Evans and Repper (2000:15) also assert that: 'Diagnosis with a mental illness commonly results in negative changes in self perception'.

As Spanswick points out, many vulnerable individuals experience mental health problems but have no discernible health problems. The sense of social isolation felt by many homeless people such as Stan may not become diagnosed with depression, although the links between poverty, unemployment and depression reveal that many people living in poverty also experience depression (Birchwood *et al.*, 1993). Such people become less and less able to extricate themselves from social exclusion (or its criteria). The process of exclusion renders them powerless and more in need of professional support, the power residing with the professional bodies. In a similar way people with learning disabilities, especially those living in the community, experience mental health problems as well as stigma arising from the negative attitudes of neighbours (Smith and Brown, 1989). The adjustments needed to move from institutionalised forms of care to community care pose a range of challenges for both the client and the professional. The evidence from Gordon *et al.* (2000) also indicates that the unemployed and those who are sick/disabled are much more likely to be categorised as poor (61 per cent). The socio-economic and demographic characteristics of poverty do not exist in isolation and, put together, local authority tenants on income support as well as disabled people stand a much higher chance of living in poverty.

People with Learning Disabilities

Studies of people with learning disabilities, including mental handicap, autism and those with visual and hearing impairment moving from institutionalised care into the community will identify with the classic work of Edgerton (1967) in terms of the stigma attached to having a disability. Living among so-called 'normal' people who may perceive others with mild learning difficulties as odd or markedly different present numerous challenges and problems which represent a form of social exclusion not considered by the SEU. The similarities between the socially excluded poor and deprived and those with learning disabilities indicate the extent to which work, or lack of it, plays a fundamental part in establishing a healthy life. The prejudices and challenges for people with learning disabilities extend beyond being looked at in the street to more fundamental issues of unemployment for the unemployables. As such, even if disabled people chose to ignore or deny their disability, the lack of day service resources limit the number of people who are able to try and normalise their lives (Sinson, 1987). A number of writers have indicated how people with a learning disability face tremendous difficulty making the transition from adolescence to adulthood because of their inability to adopt work status even in a sheltered environment (Coffield, 1987; Boston and Wite, 1987). The effects of long-term unemployment are well known but for those with learning disability resonate with other issues such as lack of money, poor self-confidence and limited experience of the social life which goes with work. One of the key issues facing staff who work with clients in community settings is managing their socially challenging behaviour in public settings. The need to provide social experiences that enable the client to deal with everyday situations such as shopping, going to the cinema/swimming pool or taking an active part in those things most of us take for granted is important, but impossible to achieve with limited staff. Lack of government funding, limited staff resources and negative public perceptions help to shape the limited experiences of those who in some cases start off socially excluded because of their impairment. People with learning disabilities are perhaps doubly vulnerable to the impact of social exclusion. First, because of the stigma, many of us have little understanding of their problems. Second, many physically and mentally disabled people are socially excluded from sharing the everyday activities others enjoy and take for granted. Finally, in terms of social exclusion, those with learning difficulties are not primarily recognised as a socially excluded group in the same way as others. This perhaps challenges us to consider not only how we conceptualise about social exclusion but, more importantly, that social exclusion may have a variety of meanings when examined from the client's perspective.

Why Are People Socially Excluded?

Explanations for the social divisions in society have been described by a number of writers notably Townsend *et al.* (1988) in terms of the genetic (survival of the fittest) explanation, as well as the behavioural and cultural (that is what they know) reasoning and the materialist justification (see Brocklehurst and Costello's chapter for a more detailed account). In 1997 the incoming Labour Government adopted a strategy that made a number of assumptions.

First, that certain social groups (particularly younger people), were marginalised from wider society primarily because of their position of being economically disadvantaged, that is, the young jobless. The Government also recognised that poverty was closely associated with other forms of deprivation such as homelessness and drug abuse, the spiral of deprivation resulting in poverty was closely shadowed by other social problems such as increased crime and various kinds of so-called social deviance, such as truancy. (Brocklehurst and Costello examine some of the key issues relating to poverty.)

Second, the connection was made between poverty and the consequences of being poor and unable to sustain the kind of life-style that enabled people to share the benefits of the new millennium. The Labour Government publicly identified the links between poverty and the vicious circle that keeps those in poverty on the margins of society. Social exclusion, as a concept, needs also to look seriously at the underlying processes which prevent people in poverty breaking out of the oppression that ties families to a life of perpetual poverty and social deprivation. This is a larger scenario that goes beyond individual issues and incorporates the notion of community care, politics and the social values/beliefs about the poor.

Finally, increases in the number of those socially excluded may be seen to stem from wider political issues, which are challenging many other Western countries. These include the move towards high-skill high-tech industries as well as increasing family breakdown. It is also clear that many basic public services, such as education and health, are failing to tackle the issues of inequality particularly where they are most needed, for example, inner city areas and deprived areas with fewer GPs, inferior shopping facilities, poor or limited housing stock and more failing schools.

Contemporary Changes

The policies of the Labour Party, which came into Government in 1997, have seen a change in approach to dealing with the health and welfare of the nation. The Government's response has been to examine and consider the wider issues surrounding inequalities. Through the development of the SEU, the Government aims to deal with closely linked problems such as poor housing, poor health and low income which result in exclusion from mainstream society for many members of the population. Setting about the task of breaking the cycle of poverty and tackling the issues of social exclusion is no easy task, but it is clearly an important goal. Consequently, the Government has set itself benchmarks, such as the eradication of child poverty by the year 2020 (Green, 2001). Initiatives developed to deal with social exclusion include the New Deal for Communities scheme which sets out to provide support for the poorest neighbourhoods through regeneration programmes that tackle issues of poor health, educational underachievement, high crime levels and poor job prospects. The essence of the initiative is the regeneration of cohesive neighbourhoods and communities. Another initiative, Sure Start, looks to improve the life prospects of younger children through family support, advice on nurturing, improved health services and access to early education. A key difference in the way these initiatives have been introduced is the approach adopted by policy developers and workers. Where other administrations and their policies have been less successful, this Government hopes to succeed because the approach is one of 'partnership' and 'working together'; gone is the traditional top-down, paternalistic approach.

Conclusion

In this chapter I have attempted to elucidate the issue that social exclusion is a process rather than a state existing in isolation to other social problems. Poverty and unemployment as key social problems should not be seen as separate entities along with a range of other mitigating factors such as low educational attainment, family breakdown and mental ill health. Moreover, as this chapter has shown, it is the interrelationships between each of the dimensions of social exclusion that help to identify how it may be prevented. I have developed the argument that, as the current pace of life in general appears to be increasing for many people, the challenges facing those who are socially excluded increase, particularly when it is recognised that many socially excluded people experience multiple deprivation. The government review (SEU, 1999a) commended the progress made by the unit in terms of focusing on the evidence it has uncovered about social exclusion. However, it also acknowledged limitations in terms of gaining access to hard evidence concerning key issues, which give rise to social exclusion discussed in this chapter, and how to tackle the interrelated nature of social exclusion. This raises the issue of whether the real challenge to policy makers is to consider the underlying social problems which give rise to social exclusion in more depth and consider making more fundamental changes in the structure of society based less on assessment outcomes and more on social experiences of the socially excluded.

References

Acheson, D. (1988) *Independent Inquiry into inequalities in health*. London: The Stationery Office.

Beaglehole, R. and Bonita, R. (1997) *Public health at the crossroads*. Cambridge, UK: Cambridge University Press.

Beynon, H. (1999) A classless society? In Beynon, H. Glavanis, P. (1999) *Patterns of social inequality*, London: Longman, 36–53.

Birchwood, M., Hallett, S. and Preston, M. (1993) Depression, demoralization and control over psychotic illness: a comparison of depressed and non depressed patients with chronic psychosis. *Psychological Medicine*, 23, 287–395.

Boston, A.M. and Wite, D. (1987) 'Inside a community': values associated with money and time. In Fineman, S. (ed.) *Unemployment: personal and social consequences*. London: Tavistock.

Coffield, F. (1987) From the celebration to the marginalisation of youth. In Cohen, G. (Ed.) *Social change and the life course*. London: Tavistock.

Costello, J. and Horne, M. (2001) Patients as teachers? An evaluative study of patients' involvement in classroom teaching. *Nurse Education in Practice*, 1, 94–102.

Edgerton, R.B. (1967) *The cloak of competence*. Berkeley: University of California Press.

Evans, J. and Repper, J. (2000) Employment, social inclusion and mental health. *Journal of Psychiatric and Mental Health Nursing*, 7, 15–24.

Giddens, A. (1997) *Sociology* (3rd edn). London: Polity Press.

Gordon, D., Adelman, L., Ashworth, K., Bradshaw, J., Levitas, R., Middleton, S., Pantazis, C., Patsios, D., Payne, S., Townsend, P. and Williams, J. (2000) *Poverty and Social Exclusion (PSE) in Britain*. York: Joseph Rowntree Foundation.

Green, L. (2001) The concept of fatalism and new Labour's role in tackling inequalities. *British Journal of Community Nursing*, 6, 3, 106–11.

Gregg, P. and Wadsworth, J. (1994) *More work in fewer households*. mimeo, London: NIESR.

Guardian (2001) Rough sleepers unit 'is fixing figures', Tania Branigan, 24 November.

Joseph Rowntree Foundation (1995) *Inquiry into income and wealth, Vol 1*. York: Joseph Rowntree Foundation.

Mason, T., Carlisle, C., Watkins, C. and Whitehead, E. (2001) *Stigma and Social Exclusion*. London: Routledge.

Milio, N. (1986) *Promoting health through public policy*. Ottawa: Canadian Public Health Association.

Moore, L.W. and Miller, M. (1999) Initiating research with doubly vulnerable populations. *Journal of Advanced Nursing*, 30, 5, 1034–40.

Petersen, A. and Lupton, D. (1996) *The new public health*. London: Sage.

SEU (Social Exclusion Unit) (1999a) *Review of the Social Exclusion Unit*. London: SEU.

SEU (Social Exclusion Unit) (1999b) *Teenage pregnancy*. London: SEU.

SEU (Social Exclusion Unit) (2000) *Young people: a report by Policy Action Team 12*. London: SEU.

SEU (Social Exclusion Unit) (2001) *Preventing Social Exclusion: a report by the Social Exclusion Unit*. London: SEU.

Sinson, J.C. (1987) *Attitudes to Down's syndrome*. London: Mental Health Foundation.

Smith, H. and Brown, H. (1989) Whose community, whose care? In Brechin, A. and Walmsley, J. *Making connections: reflecting on the lives and experiences of people with learning difficulties.* London: Hodder & Stoughton with Open University Press, 229–36.

Townsend, P., Davidson, N. and Whitehead, M. (eds) (1988) *Inequalities in health: the Black Report.* 2nd edn. London: Penguin Books.

Yin, R.K. (1994) *Case study research: design and methods.* London: Sage.

9
Public Health:
the Professional Response

MONICA HAGGART

The key points discussed in this chapter include:

- the impact of social position, relative power and health beliefs on the public's health and the role of public health nursing
- core skills and the need for change in the way that practitioners work
- some of the issues underpinning evidence-based practice in public health.

Introduction

This chapter briefly considers the arguments of the previous chapters in order to consider what the professional response can or should be in the light of the varying opinions which abound. The chapter will consider the generic professional response which may be possible particularly in terms of working together with each other and with the public. It is impossible within a single chapter to consider the role of all professionals so one professional group will be used as an exemplar for others. Public health nursing is argued to have a particular role to fulfil and the role of public health nurses as a response to public health need will be considered in more detail.

Overview

Regardless of the semantics about the nature and meaning of 'public health', the preceding chapters have highlighted a number of issues which impact upon the health of the public. The first of these factors might be argued to be the health beliefs of the public and how these are developed and manipulated by various powerful groups, to the point that the public could be perceived as being maintained in a state of ignorance while believing themselves to be well informed. Paradoxical, often unconscious, beliefs can be seen in the way that the public can simultaneously ignore the real risks to their health of the mundane, yet feel disproportionate concern over what could be construed to be abstract risks to health. For example, it is clear that we continue to smoke, consume alcohol, experience more obesity, and yet some people may refuse to travel on a long-haul flight because of the risk of deep vein thrombosis. Many people will happily travel in a car, not considering the long or short-term health consequences while berating the rail travel companies for the dangers of train travel.

King in Chapter 5 helps to understand this phenomenon in terms of the way the media construct health images. The media can often help to externalise and make threats to health more abstract. We can become enraged and taken up in these moral panics by something that has never happened and is never likely to happen to us or to anyone that we know. In this way, health and well-being can become something that is separate from ourselves, something that is out of our control, indeed it may arguably be controlled by others. Simultaneously, it is reasonable to consider a 'conspiracy theory' exists encouraged by the media who are often engaged in 'uncovering the truth' behind the most recent moral panic, leading to a general lack of trust in 'authority'. The trust is placed in the hands of those perceived to be on our side who share our lack of trust and understand our fear, that is, the media. We exchange our bestowal of power from the elected government to the unelected media. This is the power that comes from being able to shape beliefs and thinking based on whatever information the powerful body selects for us to receive. The paradox in health beliefs can then be seen in the reliance on authority, establishment and professionals and the expectation of 'protection' which results from the steady increase in institutional control over the lives of individuals where individual decision making has been eroded, as identified by Iphofen in Chapter 2.

The control of information and the feeding of a conspiracy theory play a part in maintaining vulnerable people in their situation. Many who need access to the widest possible information about their rights, health and well-being arguably have ease of access only to the pre-digested information in the media. Additionally the opinions of the rest of the public about the vulnerable groups themselves are shaped by that same media and are recognisably intolerant. Spanswick's discussions in Chapter 5 demonstrate how vulnerable people can be treated by society and how this in turn impacts on their health. Costello, in Chapter 8, takes this further by identifying the social exclusion that occurs but identifies the weakness in the government approach of dealing with outcomes rather than determinants of social exclusion.

In Chapter 3 Brocklehurst and Costello focus on the failure of 'medicine' to make any real impression on health and well-being, particularly in groups affected by social disadvantage. The reasons for persisting health inequality are identified as life-style and its impact on health, the impact of sustained social inequality on mental health and the effects of powerful groups limiting individual opportunities for health. These factors can be related to a lack of power and perhaps to some degree lack of control over life events and arguably the absence of social support in promoting change.

Costello *et al.* in Chapter 4, while focusing on ethnic minority groups also highlight a generalised oppression and wielding of power over the powerless. The imperative for everyone to look the same, wear the same clothes, be absent of facial hair at certain ages or in certain occupations, to behave in the same way and to believe the same things brings with it the acceptance into or rejection from the mainstream group. It is in this mainstream group that people can expect to be protected, educated, employed and have their health needs met. When outside of the mainstream group for whatever reason, access to these 'privileges' is made more difficult.

The preceding chapters highlight the failure of the establishment (and professionals as the representatives of the establishment) to create the kind of structure within society that promotes health. Indeed, as Illich (1975) argued, it may be that professionals have in the past been part of the problem. Iphofen in Chapter 2 makes this point and identifies how epidemiology has failed to inform the public about health status partly because of the way that statistics are collated and reported as percentages and averages across groups and communities. In this way people don't recognise themselves or their real lives within the science, thus contributing to the lack of trust, alienation and disengagement in health matters. Horne in Chapter 7 offers some alternative means of identifying health needs with more narrative approaches that have meaning for people because of their origins within their real lives. These chapters identify a need for a different way of working with communities if indeed we are to improve the health of the public. What we are left to explore now is how professionals should respond to the needs outlined. The remainder of this chapter is devoted to outlining some of the core professional responsibilities, particularly focusing on public health nursing as one group of professionals who can be argued to have something to offer the new public health approaches.

The Professional Response

Two historical events influenced the development of a gradual culture shift which began after the Second World War and before the inception of the NHS. This shift is recognised through consumer activity, personal acquisitiveness and aspirations to increasing affluence. Le Fanu (1999) indicates the not entirely coincidental major advances in medical science that occurred during this period. These advances may have contributed to a general feeling of invincibility, but importantly higher and higher expectations from life in general and medicine in particular. This cultural shift and the overall philosophy of life that it engendered was seized upon by the Government in the early 1980s in its neo-liberalist drive to reduce the 'nanny state', reorganise health and other public services along business lines and to promote health as a product of an individual's 'life-style choices'.

Halliday (2002) highlights how the British Government's direction in the 1980s was one of individualism as well as the 'lifestylism' and victim blaming that accompanied it. The World Health Organisation (WHO, 1984) recognised the phenomenon of victim blaming when it identified the potential for health programmes to be inappropriately directed at individuals rather than tackling the fundamental economic and social influences upon health. The World Health Organisation in the meantime was taking a somewhat different approach from which many British practitioners and academics were taking their inspiration. The Black Report (DHSS, 1980) was studiously ignored, but the1980s also gave birth to the Ottawa Charter (1986) and the courageous Ashton and Seymour (1988) treatise on developing the 'New Public Health' – courageous because it was somewhat against the British tide in outlining the social conditions which were giving rise to the widespread health problems, recognising that all public services had a responsibility for health and that new ways of working must be designed in order to meet the needs.

Ashton and Seymour (1988) tie the 'new public health' very closely with the Ottawa Charter, which stresses the necessity to:

> Build public policies which support health
> Create supportive environments
> Strengthen community action
> Develop personal skills
> Re-orientate health services

Ashton and Seymour (1988) highlight the commitment in public health work to power sharing, demystification of knowledge and a social contract with communities.

Working in Partnership with the Community – Building Social Capital

Ashton (2000) identifies the need for what he refers to as the 'new citizenship' to be a key issue for government and for local changes to a more participative approach when working with communities. The word 'citizenship' is something that has infiltrated current government language and, if misunderstood, might even resemble community manipulation, identified by Arnstein (1969) in her discussions of the potential for community involvement. However, Ashton is persuasive in his argument that societies, not least British society, are becoming increasingly fragmented and fractured. He suggests that this is evidenced by ever-increasing intolerance, blaming of others, war and hatred, all of which are common features of modern society. Some common strands to these elements which Ashton identifies as found in many societies are:

- loss of a shared ethical framework and set of common values
- sense of powerlessness
- loss of sense of community and control
- fear of a changing world
- jealousy, envy and pride
- poor leadership in many quarters
- lack of accountability of our institutions, and of powerful professional and other groups
- lack of adequate systems to mediate between conflicting groups' interests and needs.

Ashton claims that tolerance and co-existence are key elements of the 'new citizenship' which can only be founded on mutual respect and recognition of interdependence. This is work that must involve everybody, and therefore participation and partnership between people is the life-blood of competent communities.

Participation underpins social integration, the development of social networks, and the overall provision of social support which promotes self-esteem and perceived security (Gottlieb, 1987), as well as social connectedness (Berkman, 2000), the absence of which is associated with higher levels of disease (Berkman, 2000; Kawachi, 2000). Working with people in a way that recognises and works on their agenda, encourages and facilitates their contributions, and works to build social networks could be argued to be working in some way to build social support and social cohesion in communities. This way of working achieves what is described by some as social capital. Social capital may be described as a concept and therefore difficult to encapsulate but could be identified as demonstrating the features of a social network that enables people to act together more effectively for mutual benefit.

The notion of social capital is not without its critics. Hawe and Shiell (2000) recognise the value of the relational aspects of this way of working but believe that the political aspects have been underexplored, and Adler and Kwon (2001) identify how the social capital of one community may be achieved at the expense of another. Mackian (2002) suggests that we must address how some of the organisations within which professionals reside build their own social capital as this has an impact on their ability to engage with communities effectively. Others, however, testify to the notion of positive effects of social capital on welfare in general (for example, Coleman, 1990; Putnam, 1995; Blane, Brunner and Wilkinson, 1996).

Working in partnership and participation, then, is a two-way process (Mackian, 2002) which, in itself, impacts on people's well-being because these are interactive concepts. Professionals working in this way can act as conduits for received information, expertise and knowledge from communities and ensure that this is accessible to policy makers at all levels, informing needs assessments and impacting upon social policies. This would involve all professionals working within a community viewing themselves certainly as potential advocates for that community by truly listening, sharing and communicating. It is proposed in this work that, by increasing the levels of participation, people within the community are more likely to feel that they have a stake, care what happens to their community and view themselves as an important part of it.

Inter-agency Alliances

Post-modern societies are complex and require a more sophisticated approach than has been hitherto demonstrated by public services in order to develop the mutual working that Ashton's (2000) new citizenship requires. The partnership working previously discussed must extend to agencies themselves, that is, inter-agency collaboration. Funnell *et al.* (1995) identify five key features of 'alliance building' which are related to benefits from both the process and the product.

1   *Commitment* – a shared commitment to the goals of the partnership

2   *Community involvement* – partnership with the community in all activities of the alliance

3   *Communication* – partners share relevant information and commit to simplicity, openness and honesty

4   *Joint working* – implies equal ownership and appropriate input from each partner

5   *Accountability* – evaluation is built into alliance work and results are used constructively.

Fundamental to these aims is that collaborative working is greater than the sum of its parts; by working together, a creativity is generated that produces something new. That 'something new' should be a more honest and open approach to identifying need and a willingness to take risks based on the power that arises from working with others on a shared vision.

Current government administration seems to recognise the advantages of collaborative working and have outlined the importance of 'joined-up working' throughout all their literature on social exclusion (for example DoH, 2000a, 2001a). Costello in his chapter identifies this as key to successful working in preventing and resolving social exclusion. This is now made more tangible by the formation of Local Strategic Partnerships (LSPs) (DoH, 2000b) which 'will bring together those who deliver or commission different services together with recipients of the service. It also ensures that other local partnerships know how they fit into the picture'. Over time these LSPs will prepare community strategies and presumably apply for associated funding. Quite how this will work in practice when most members of these partnerships work as employees of the very organisations that they may be pressing for further resources, remains uncertain. However, within most codes of practice there are clauses which identify the duty of the professional to advocate for the client at all times, and practitioners would do well to use this more often as their *raison d'être*.

Only time will tell whether the government agenda is intended as a real attempt to reduce social exclusion or simply to give that impression. Professionals in the meantime have a mandate to work with communities in this way and there is a real opportunity to provide a bottom-up approach to improving the public's health. First the joint working between agencies and local populations, if authentic, is likely to result in an informed population who will be able to take responsibility for actions and outcomes and seek real causes and solutions for problems, rather than simply lay blame. Second, if demand arises from an informed population who recognise their interdependence, any provision is much more likely to meet the need.

Public Health Nursing

Public health nursing is not new but has been discussed in the British nursing literature almost as a new profession. Internationally, however, public health nursing has a long history. In Canada, Finland, Sweden (and arguably in Ireland), for example, public health nurses work in very similar ways to extant British health visitors (Kahn and Landes, 1993). Caraher and McNab (1996) argue that British public health should be working at a broad level, looking to identify the determinants of health and reduce the impact of social inequalities. They caution, however, that public health nursing should have a clear idea about what the role encompasses. In the USA, public health nursing, according to Kuss *et al.* (1997) encapsulates the following concepts:

- community empowerment
- public health nursing history and nursing education
- core public health functions
- environmental forces
- caring
- interdisciplinary collaboration
- community partnership.

There are recognisable areas where public health nurses will work with other agencies and disciplines and some of these core concepts have already been discussed. Each professional response will include the specialist skills associated with the particular profession. These will now be discussed in relation to public health nursing, and the question is posed: what additional skills do public health nurses contribute to improving the public health?

Caring

The term 'caring' is emotive and over-used within the academic literature that describes what nurses do. Kuss *et al.* (1997) identify it as an underpinning concept, although it is not clear how it may impact on public health. However, it is not so over-used in the medical, social and epidemiological world of public health. Phillips (1993) suggests that caring should be viewed as a fundamental part of healing but not necessarily the polar opposite of cure. She suggests that caring requires the care giver to be responsive to the needs of the person being cared for, which involves: 'skilled assessment, planning, action and evaluation of the implications and nuances of all these factors'. The much misunderstood, often criticised and equally over-used concept of 'holism' has been one that many claim lies at the heart of nursing and identifies nursing as a therapeutic force in itself. Holism is not a set of therapies or activities but is a philosophical approach that drives the way practitioners practice. Laura and Heaney (1990) suggest that within a holistic framework issues of health and disease are viewed as features of the complex interplay between the whole person and the total environment.

Caring is often discussed only in terms of nursing within a hospital setting with people who are ill and therefore categorised as patients. However, much of the literature around the 'new' nursing identifies outcomes of caring that are about improving the human condition. Brykczyńska (1992), for example, highlights how caring in nursing can serve to reduce the spiritual distress that people encounter when life loses its meaningfulness and hope. Barber (1991) identifies clearly and poignantly the therapeutic potential of caring in terms of 'healing' which he identifies to mean long-term personal growth.

Brykczyńska (1992) identifies caring as an elusive concept which must be analysed in a professional setting to avoid defining it simply as an emotional response. She explores the five specific constructs of professional caring identified by Roach (1985) as *compassion, competence, confidence, conscience* and *commitment*. Compassion may be identified as the emotional response which involves putting yourself in the position of others. Competence in the practice of nursing (whatever the specialism) involves an 'inquiring mind and a searching heart'. Roach (1985) describes compassion without competence as a meaningless, if not harmful, intrusion into another person's life. Confidence may be viewed alternatively as assertion, while conscience is the level of moral integrity which underpins the trust that nurses are privileged to receive from the public. Finally, commitment describes the nurse's commitment to the person which is not a passing phenomenon or emotion which lasts just as long as the person is a 'patient' or part of a caseload but which identifies their needs as important, to be addressed for as long as necessary, so identifying the long-term nature of caring.

From these constructs it is clear that caring has a part to play in working with people at a public health level. It is not just about an emotional response to people who are ill, it is about working in a specific way that values people as persons and in so doing helps them to value themselves. This can be seen as connected to Antonovsky's (1984, 1996) salutogenic model (discussed in more detail below) in that the activity of caring in this context could be seen to work to increase the sense of coherence that can be held by an individual but equally could be discerned in a community. Even from this brief discussion we can see that nursing has many skills to bring to the new public health.

Public health nursing may therefore be identified as a specific branch of community nursing which brings all aspects of the person and potential influences on their health together with all aspects of the environment that they live in. It brings together the unique skills of nursing to ensure that 'healing' in its fullest sense can take place. Arguably, however, the nurse who works with the public's health has specific additional educational needs in terms of social frameworks of health and working with vulnerable populations.

Health Promotion

Promoting health is a key principle of the new public health, according to Ashton and Seymour (1988). This may make sociologists throw up their hands in horror as it smacks of hidden agendas and manipulation. However, this of course depends upon the approach to health promotion that is espoused, as models of health promotion often reflect the particular philosophies of health on which they are based. Antonovsky's model is considered to be a suitable model for public health nursing as it is sufficiently flexible to be used at an individual or collective level and it takes an unashamedly holistic and humanistic stance.

Antonovsky (1984, 1996) calls his model the 'salutogenic' model of health promotion, arguing that most other models adopt a pathogenic orientation. This dichotomously classifies people as either sick or not, and in order to avoid sickness, we must avoid the risk factors. The public then is encouraged to protect themselves from these 'risk factors' through immunisation and ever-increasing levels of medication. They are encouraged to see health as outside of themselves and within the power of others (Illich, 1975). Antonovsky takes the stance that the human system is inherently flawed, subject to unavoidable entropic (health threatening) processes and unavoidable final death. We must, according to Antonovsky, explore what factors actively promote health. He proposed the Sense of Coherence (SOC) construct, which leads each of us to see life as more or less comprehensible, manageable and meaningful. The strength of any individual's SOC is a significant factor in facilitating the movement towards health. Further, the strength of the SOC is shaped by three kinds of life experiences, that is, consistency, underload–overload balance and participation in socially valued decision making.

One major advantage of Antonovsky's model is that it distances health promotion from the medically moulded health education and screening approaches. He argues that strengthening the SOC is about people having meaningful positions in society, being valued within their social group and having meaningful occupations. This would involve those working towards improvements in public health, changing or working to change structures which oppress people and leave them with little sense of purpose, importance or self-esteem.

If, as seems often to be the case, we define public health solely according to the medical model, that is, specific disease prevention targets, screening, infectious disease control and the like, we would be correct to question whether there was a place here for nursing. However, it is now generally recognised that people's needs, particularly in the fractured communities that currently exist in Britain, are greater than simply the avoidance of disease. The needs, certainly in Antonovsky's terms, can be identified as more to do with developing mutual respect for the human condition and development of self-esteem and confidence in the ability to cope with life and each other in a complex world. The role of the nurse can be discerned within this approach to the promotion of the public's health. In the same way that nurses work with individuals, then nurses can work with communities in a mutual way to recognise people's skills, to build on them in bringing people together to promote their own and others' health.

Current UK government administration clearly see a role for public health, as is demonstrated in the plethora of documents that outline an increasingly complex approach to reducing inequalities, renewing neighbourhoods and ultimately improving the public health. The Chief Medical Officer's report on strengthening the public health function (DoH, 2000c) recognises the role for all nurses as being among several professional groups working at a strategic level in public health. It is not however the business of this chapter to define a series of tasks identifying what public health nurses do, rather it is to identify how they might do them in a way that can be identified specifically as public health approaches.

Working for Health not Sickness

Nursing theorists over the last few decades have developed a vision of what nursing can achieve when practiced more autonomously (for example, Benner, 1984; Benner and Wrubel, 1992; Ersser, 1988). The realities of working as a nurse within the restrictions of the powerful medical model, however, have not allowed the required freedom to develop the vision. Where this freedom to think differently has been encouraged, there is evidence of improvement in people's lives. For example, Pearson *et al.* (1992) demonstrate that patients in a nurse-led unit compared to a medically-led unit had reduced dependency and readmission rates and increased patient satisfaction.

Public health nursing within the framework espoused in this chapter clearly involves taking some of the core skills of nursing and using them 'outside the box' of the traditional parameters which focus on sickness not health. It involves working from a health perspective and working alongside people in a way designed to be health enhancing rather than health damaging. Nursing can work to maintain people in sickness or to help them towards health, according to Macleod Clarke (1993). Macleod Clarke identifies two kinds of nursing. The one, 'sick nursing' is where care is determined by the diagnosis or problem, care is *administered* to the patient, expertise and knowledge *owned* by the nurse and other professionals and decision making is *dominated* by the professional rather than the patient or client. The other, a health model of nursing, she argues, focuses on *maximising the client's potential* for health and independence, builds on people's *existing* knowledge and experience, helps them to become more *autonomous* and empowers them to take *responsibility* for their own health. She identifies clearly that the kind of nursing that is undertaken is dependent upon the nature of the interactions.

This is something that we already know from the work of people like Marteau and Baum (1984) who demonstrated how physicians' attitudes to diabetes impacted upon their perceptions of the benefits of treatment, therefore the action taken and ultimately the patient outcome. Weinberger *et al.* (1984) also demonstrated how the stronger a physician's belief in the efficacy of blood glucose control, the more likely patients were to achieve near normal blood glucose levels. Marteau and Johnston (1990) suggest that based on these and other studies the beliefs and behaviours of health professionals are potential targets for change in maximising patient's health outcomes.

Nurses' professional attitudes, that is, the *way* they work with people, will impact on the way that people view themselves and their human potential, which in turn will impact on their health. These interactions and the philosophies that underpin them are a function of the power structures within which nurses work. These approaches reflect a dominant medical ideology and the authoritarian structure which they support, and while this prevails, a move from 'sick nursing' to 'health nursing' may be too difficult for many nurses either in hospital or in primary care.

Public health nursing, if it is to encapsulate many of the issues raised in this book, is as much about process as product. Its focus is working with people at a collective level, building on their strengths and abilities, taking into account the many, varied and complex issues such as, for example, holism, environment, politics, class. Public health nursing harnesses the core skills of nursing and extends them into the arena of working with people who are well, coping with, and managing their lives as success- fully as they can. It is also about participating with people in bringing about change to those situations which will improve the circumstances, social capital and potential for health of all members of the community, and above all recognising their interdependence. Two key questions remain. How do we know it will make a difference, and is it possible within the current and proposed NHS structures? These questions will be addressed in the next sections.

Opposing Paradigms

Within clinical governance there is a laudable drive to develop nursing as an evidence-based profession. The evidence in question is generally research, but within nursing generally and certainly public health nursing this is not as simple as it seems. Oakley (2001) recognises what she calls a 'paradigm war' between the research methods which are traditionally used to observe the implementation, history and impact of social interventions and those which are used to assess clinical interventions. Biological determinism, individualism, isolation and blame remain the contested, but still dominant, ideology in health care. The reasons for this dominance are outside the remit of this chapter and are discussed more than adequately in other publications, for example, RUHBC (1989). Arguably, a factor in this dominance is the culture shift which sees death as the final taboo, to be avoided at all costs. Examples of this attitude can be seen in such documents as *Saving Lives. Our Healthier Nation* (DoH, 1999a) where targets are set for the major diseases and the emphasis is on reducing deaths from the 'killer' diseases. We measure success by avoidance of death, regardless of the quality of life that results for those 'treated' individuals, and continues untended for others.

Health and its determinants are a complex interplay of many factors but are traditionally subsumed under the power of a body of professionals whose expertise lies within illness. Their success in dealing with illness when it occurs, and even of preventing certain specific illnesses, is well documented. However, this does not make the medical establishment experts in health, because at the risk of using a cliché, health is about more than the absence of disease, it is not within the expertise of the medical establishment. However even within medicine there is a growing recognition of the importance of the psycho-social context and its impact on people's lives, although many forces operate to retain the illness/treatment focus of research.

Public pressure arises from the culture of professional expectation (arguably arising from an over-professionalisation of everyday life from birth to death and everything in between) and the avoidance of death at whatever cost. This is translated into pressure on the medical establishment to save life (the more spectacularly the better), to give answers to thus far unanswerable questions, and then successfully to treat all illnesses. We can measure that success by the fact that the patient is still alive. This public perception is translated via the medical establishment but, importantly, also via the media into political pressure. A general political drive results via the power-base of research funding agencies but also provider agencies which seem to value only that which results in reduced mortality rates. If success is about the avoidance of death, then we simply need to measure the reduction in the number of deaths to demonstrate how successful we are!

Increasing knowledge of the body and how it works means that we must break down understanding into its smallest parts and exclude as far as possible all external factors (without considering the possibility that it is those outside factors which exert a great deal of influence). Randomised Controlled Trials (RCTs) are the 'gold standard' of research and can be argued to attract much of the research funding as well as wielding the most power in terms of changing policy. RCTs are a very useful research method for discovering if a certain factor leads to a particular outcome. This however leads to a plethora of evidence for the efficacy of particular medical treatments or influences on certain medical conditions. Notwithstanding, it also leads to a paucity of research (other than small scale) about issues or interventions which may impact on people's overall health over the long term. Arguably, much research is turned down for funding because it does not meet the rigorous standards and criteria set and applied by the research funding bodies. Cutliffe (2001) argues that there is greater acceptance of the epistemological and methodological beliefs of the medical model than more qualitative approaches, suggesting that this leads, to a hegemony of randomised controlled trials. Leininger (1992) also identifies the additional difficulties encountered when trying to gain funding for qualitative research. Nursing has no large-scale funding research body, nurse researchers have to submit to the medical research funding bodies and therefore have to meet the criteria that are set. This has the potential, over a period of time, to drive nursing research down a bio-medical route and suppress research which is not bio-medically driven. It will be interesting to see if the increased nursing research funding announced in 2002, as well as the new committee to advise on the future funding of research (Scott, 2002), will make a difference to this situation.

Using What Evidence We Have

The public health nurse cannot change the research funding bodies or their criteria of acceptance single-handedly and has a duty, with all other professionals, to do more good than harm and to address questions of effectiveness through reliable evaluation methods. A route must be found through this evidence jungle to continue to work for the promotion of people's health. This might be achieved in two ways. First, searching, finding, interpreting, evaluating and utilising effectively, research that has already been undertaken. Horne in Chapter 7 discusses the need for a sound understanding and expertise in epidemiological traditions but also combined with that, the need to be in touch with the community in order to record the reality of their situation. Second, by designing appropriate evaluation studies of both the process and the outcome of any proposed intervention. These activities demand skills of systematic searching but also of interpretation and evaluation.

Oakley (2001) identifies how policy planning is rarely informed by research findings in a linear way, even when the policy makers commissioned the research in the first place. There are many pressures on policy makers who will ultimately seek a way through the planning process which appears most logical and fits within the frameworks with which they are familiar. The public health nurse can, having identified and evaluated the research, help policy planners put the research into that framework. For example, demonstrating the link between studies which demonstrate that social support leads to reduction of stress and studies which identify stress as a factor in suppression of the immune system leading to increased incidence of illness. By linking evidence in this way, the public health nurse may not be presenting an incontrovertible argument but is at least presenting a body of evidence which may help policy planners to question and perhaps reassess their priorities.

Evaluation of proposed interventions will involve two fundamental elements of identifying and ranking the criteria against which to measure and then gathering the evidence that will make it possible to assess whether the criteria are being met. Maxwell (1984) identifies five evaluation criteria which have been contested as to their value outside of health *care* services but despite that are well used within health promotion (Table 9.1). They do seem to offer an opportunity for the needs of policy planners to be brought together with the needs of a community in assessing the value of an intervention.

Table 9.1   Criteria for evaluation

Effectiveness	The extent to which aims and objectives are met (and in public health interventions it is assumed that the public have been involved in devising the aims and objectives)
Appropriateness	Relevance to need. Again the assumption underlying this when applied to public health is that the public were involved in identifying the need
Acceptability	To the people concerned and society at large
Equity	Whether it provides equally for those with equal needs. This includes an evaluation of accessibility of the service to different groups
Efficiency	Involves some calculation of relative costs and benefits. (The public should be involved in identifying the benefits for them which can later be interpreted into the language of the policy planner)

Source: Maxwell (1984).

This kind of evaluation is clearly part of the participatory and collaborative process that is public health nursing. Within the resource-limited health environment that we have, there is a duty that is incumbent on all practitioners, whether medical, nursing or other professional, to assess the value of activities intended to improve the lives of the people with whom we work. The problems that exist within the system of research funding, as outlined earlier, cannot be used as a reason not to develop evidence for practice, whatever that practice is. This can of course be done while still working for change. Public health nurses can be at the forefront of designing rigorous research which will demonstrate to funding bodies that there are different forms of evidence all of which have a place in developing the knowledge base.

The Case for Public Health Nursing

Many nurses have skills which enable them to incorporate public health principles into their existing work and indeed this is what the Government is keen for nurses to do (for example, DoH, 2001a). SNMAC (1995) similarly suggest that all nurses, midwives and health visitors have a contribution to make to the public health, citing infection control and accident prevention among other areas where they might use these skills. However, nurses using skills related to public health as part of their work is not essentially public health nursing which, in order to merit the title, must at least espouse the basic principles of public health. According to Turton *et al.* (2000) these can be viewed as: equity, collaboration, participation and strengthening community action.

The UKCC (now the Nursing and Midwifery Council) created more than one tangled mess of titles in its lifetime with little consideration for the implications for practice. They seem to have achieved this again with the arbitrary use of the title 'public health nurse' attached to the health visitor title since 1997. Having been given the title, are health visitors indeed the public health nurses of the future? That really depends on them.

The principles of health visiting were established by the Council for the Education and Training of Health Visitors (CETHV, 1974) but have been revisited and are deemed to be equally appropriate for today (Twinn and Cowley, 1992). They are:

- Search for health needs.
- Stimulate awareness of health needs.
- Influence policies affecting health.
- Facilitate health enhancing activities.

These principles, when analysed, can be seen to encapsulate some, if not all, of the issues and principles of public health discussed above. The deficit within the principles is that they discuss what will be done rather than how it will be done, whereas in public health terms the product is a variable that is dependent upon the process.

Public health nursing as it has been discussed may have a slightly different emphasis to other discussions that are available, as interpretations on the varied role of public health nurses vary. This chapter explores a distinct nursing focus to public health practice, recognising it as one element within the public health system. This nursing focus may be a problem for some health visitors who are keen to shed the notion of the need for nursing as an underpinning of health visiting. However, it is argued here that the core skills of nursing bring to public health something that is unique and can be recognised distinctly as *nursing*. Other health visitors wish to remain firmly within the extant primary care system, undertaking much the same work which is undoubtedly not community focused, applying interventions without community participation and arguably operating from a very limited framework of collaboration. This again is their prerogative, but is too limiting to be recognised as public health nursing by any interpretation of the definition(s) of public health nursing.

There is clearly a drive for health visitors to be viewed as public health nurses, but in order to achieve this there need to be changes in three main areas, that is, policy support, context of working and education. There appears to be no real support in policy for any nurses working in the way outlined above. However, with a willingness to be creative, strategic clinical leaders within primary care trusts could work with health visitors and the community in changing the way that health visitors work. This may involve removing them from the primary care equation and identifying a specific public health division which has a clear role in reducing inequalities in health. Primary care in the way that it is currently defined in Britain is not an appropriate setting for public health nurses. The power base within primary medical care is one which is medically dominated with a focus on illness, treatment and individual behaviour. While recognising medical care is an important element of the public's well-being, it is not the central focus of public health.

The education of health visitors, of course, fits within the framework of the work that health visitors are expected to do. There are clear demands for health visitors to become at least more public health focused (DoH, 1999, 2001b) and education will have to change along with this. The English National Board for Nursing Midwifery and Health Visiting (ENB, 2000) found health visitor education wanting in this respect, although the UKCC (1994) demanded learning outcomes relevant to public health for health visitors in the programme leading to the qualification of Community Specialist Practitioner Health Visiting – Public Health

Nursing. Universities face the twin pressures of meeting the UKCC guidance and the demands from practice to equip health visitors with the skills that they need for the 'real world', that is, the work they will actually be undertaking in practice. Health visitors appear to be the natural professional to hold the title of 'public health nurse', however they may have to let go of some things that they hold dear and apply pressure to put in place the structure and policies which will enable them to carry out their work.

Conclusion

This chapter has argued that the professional response to the needs of the public in pursuit of health clearly has to change. The current over-professionalised, paternalistic way of working drives people into feeling that they are unable to manage their health and life without professional intervention (Illich, 1975; Macleod Clark, 1993). Western societies can be seen to be fragmented, fractured and alienated from themselves (Ashton, 2000) and it is this to which practitioners who work with communities must respond. The core of this response is suggested in this chapter to incorporate a more inclusive way of working which involves a more 'joined up' way of working. Practitioners must join up with the communities which they serve but also with each other. These can be viewed to be the core skills of community working.

Each practitioner group has specialist skills to add to what are viewed here as core, and this chapter has highlighted public health nursing for particular attention.

Nightingale's (1893) notion of a nursing 'proper' and health nursing may be a notion that is usefully considered even today. There is a distinction between nursing the sick and nursing the well in order to prevent 'sickness', and this may be clearly distinguished in public health nursing. Public health nursing arose from the same imperative that gave birth to the new public health and is clearly outlined in this chapter as a role that draws on the best principles of nursing whereby the product is a function of the process. It is proposed in this chapter that public health nursing is a strategic combination of holistic caring, health promotion, advocacy through interpretation of data, partnership, collaboration and working for health not sickness.

Whoever is to be given the mantle of public health nursing, whether this is a whole profession or a disparate group of nurses working in a particular way, they must develop an evidence-based structure. This will involve them in collating and connecting data to advocate for clients and communities. It would also involve developing rigorous research strategies that stay true to the holistic foundation of their work, but which equally command credibility from the powerful organisations which are given the public's trust in terms of determining research funding.

Finally, to realise the goals of public health nursing, primary care trusts must demonstrate the courage that will be required to maintain the public health nurse outside of the structure of primary medical care. This may be by establishing clear and separate public health divisions and locating within that division the key professionals who will work collaboratively across boundaries, offering the opportunity for a true primary *health* care system.

References

Adler, P.S. and Kwon, S.W. (2001) Social Capital: Prospects for a New Concept. *Academy of Management Review*, 27, 1, 17–40.

Antonovsky, A. (1984) The Sense of Coherence as a Determinant of Health. In Matarazzo, J.P. (ed.) *Behavioural Health*. New York: Wiley.

Antonovsky, A. (1996) The Salutogenic Model as a Theory Guide to Health. *Health Promotion International* 11, 1, 11–18.

Arnstein, S. (1969) A Ladder of Participation. *Journal of the American Planning Association*, 35, 4, 214–19.

Ashton, J.R. (2000) Governance, Health & the New Citizenship. Inaugural Lecture at Liverpool John Moores University, North West Public Health Observatory. http://www.nwpho.org.uk. accessed 3 January 2002.

Ashton, J. and Seymour, H. (1988) *The New Public Health*. Milton Keynes: Open University Press.

Barber, P. (1991) Caring; The Nature of a Therapeutic Relationship. In Perry, A. and Jolley, M. (1991) (eds) *Nursing: A Knowledge Base for Practice*, London: Edward Arnold.

Benner, P. (1984) *From Novice to Expert*. New York and Menlo Park, CA: Addison Wesley.

Benner, P. and Wrubel, J. (1992) *The Primacy of Caring*. Menlo Park, CA: Addison Wesley.

Berkman, L.F. (2000) Social Networks and Health. The Bonds That Heal. In Tarlov, I. and St Peter, R.F. (2000) *The Society & Population Health. A Reader*. New York: The New Press.

Blane, D., Brunner, E. and Wilkinson R. (1996) *Health & Social Organisations*. London: Routledge.

Brykczyńska, G. (1992) Caring – A Dying Art? In Jolley, M. and Bryczyńska, G. (1992) *Nursing Care. The Challenge to Change*. London: Edward Arnold.

Caraher, M. and McNab, M. (1996) The Public Health Nursing Role: An Overview of Future Trends. *Nursing Standard*, 10, 51, 44–8.

CETHV (Council for the Education & Training of Health Visitors) (1974) *The Principles of Health Visiting*. London: CETHV.

Coleman, J.S. (1990) *Foundations of Social Theory*. Cambridge, MA: Harvard University Press.

Cutliffe, J. (2001) The Long and Winding Road: Obtaining Funding for Qualitative Research Proposals. *Nurse Researcher*, 9, 1, 52–62.

DoH (Department of Health) (2001a) *Inequalities in Health. From Vision to Reality*. London: Department of Health.

DoH (Department of Health) (2001b) *Health Visitor Practice Development Resource Park*. London: Department of Health.

DoH (Department of Health) (2000a) *Tackling Social Exclusion*. London: Social Exclusion Unit.

DoH (Department of Health) (2000b) *A New Commitment to Neighbourhood Renewal. A National Strategy Action Plan*. London: Social Exclusion Unit.

DoH (Department of Health) (2000c) *The Report of the Chief Medical Officer's Project to Strengthen the Public Health Function.* London: HMSO.

DoH (Department of Health) (1999a) *Saving Lives. Our Healthier Nation.* London: The Stationery Office.

DoH (Department of Health) (1999) *Making a Difference. Strengthening the Nursing, Midwifery and Health Visiting Contribution to Health and Health Care.* London: Department of Health.

DHSS (1980) *Report on the Inequalities in Health (The Black Report).* London: HMSO.

ENB (English Board for Nursing, Midwifery and Health Visiting) (2000) *Evaluation of the Developing Specialist Practitioner Role in the Context of Public Health.* London: English National Board.

Ersser, S. (1988) Nursing Beds and Nursing Therapy. In Pearson, A. (1988) *Primary Nursing.* London: Chapman & Hall.

Funnell, R., Oldfield, K. and Speller, V. (1995) *Towards Healthier Alliances.* London: Health Education Authority.

Gottlieb, B.H.(1987) Using Social Support to Protect and Promote Health. *Journal of Primary Prevention,* 8, 49–70.

Halliday, M. (2002) Practicing Health for All in the UK. In Adams, L., Amos, M. and Munro, J. (2002) *Promoting Health. Policies & Practice.* London: Sage Publications.

Hawe, P. and Shiell, A. (2000) Social Capital and Health Promotion. A Review. *Social Science & Medicine,* 51, 871–85.

Illich, I. (1975) *Medical Nemesis. Limits to Medicine.* London: Marion Boyars.

Kahn, M. and Landes, R. (1993) The Role of the Public Health Nurse. A Review of the International Literature. Occasional Paper 2. Salford: Public Health Research and Resource Centre.

Kawachi, I. (2000) Social Cohesion and Health. In Tarlov, I. and St Peter, R.F. (2000) *The Society & Population Health. A Reader.* New York: The New Press.

Kuss, T., Proulx-Girouard, L., Lovitt, S. and Kennelly, P. (1997) A Public Health Nursing Model. *Public Health Nursing,* 14, 2, 81–91.

Laura, R.S. and Heaney, S. (1990) *The Philosophical Foundations of Health Education.* London: Routledge.

Le Fanu, J. (1999) *The Rise and Fall of Modern Medicine.* London: Little Brown & Co.

Leininger, M. (1992) Current Issues, Problems and Trends to Advance Qualitative Paradigmatic Research Methods For the Future. *Qualitative Health Research,* 9, 2, 163–5.

Mackian, S. (2002) Complex Cultures. Rereading the Story About Health and Social Capital. *Critical Social Policy,* 22, 2, 203–25.

Macleod Clarke, J. (1993) From Sick Nursing to Health Nursing: Evolution or Revolution. In Wilson Barnett, J. and Macleod Clark, J. (1993) *Research in Health Promotion and Nursing.* Basingstoke: Macmillan – now Palgrave.

Martau, T.M. and Baum, J.D. (1984) Doctor's Views on Diabetes. *Archives of Disease in Childhood,* 59, 566–70.

Marteau, T.M. and Johnston, M. (1990) Health Professionals: A Source of Variance in Health Outcomes. *Psychology and Health,* 5, 47–58.

Maxwell, R.J. (1984) Quality Assessment in Health Care. *British Medical Journal,* 288, 166–203.

Nightingale, F. (1893) *Sick Nursing and Health Nursing.* In Seymour, L. (1954) *Selected writings of Florence Nightingale.* New York: Macmillan – now Palgrave.

Oakley, A. (2001) Evaluating Health Promotion: Methodological Diversity. In Oliver, S. and Peersman, G. (2001) *Using Research for Effective Health Promotion* Buckingham: Open University Press.

Ottawa Charter for Health Promotion (1986) An International Conference on Health Promotion: The Move Towards a New Public Health. Ottawa: World Health Organisation.

Pearson, A., Punton, S. and Durant, I. (1992) *Nursing Beds. An Evaluation of the Effects of Therapeutic Nursing.* London: Scutari Press.

Phillips, P. (1993) A deconstruction of caring. *Journal of Advanced Nursing,* 18, 1554–8.

Putnam, R.D. (1995) Bowling alone – America's Declining Social Capital. *Journal of Democracy,* 6, 1, 65–78.

Roach, S.M. (1985) A Foundation for Nursing Ethics. In Carmi, A. and Schneider, S. (eds) (1985) *Nursing Law and Ethics.* Berlin: Springer-Verlag.

RUHBC (Regional Unit in Health and Behavioural Change) (1989) *Changing the Public Health* Chichester: John Wiley & Sons.

Scott, G. (2002) Funding Boost is on the Way for Nursing Research. *Nursing Standard*, 16, 36, 6.

SNMAC (Standing Nursing & Midwifery Advisory Committee) (1995) *Making it Happen. Public Health, the Contribution, Role and Development of Nurses, Midwives and Health Visitors*. London: Department of Health.

Turton, P., Peckham, S. and Taylor, P. (2000) *Public Health in Primary Care*. In Craig, P.M. and Lindsay, G.M. (2000) *Nursing for Public Health. Population Based Care*. Edinburgh: Churchill Livingstone.

Twinn, S. and Cowley, S. (1992) *The Principles of Health Visiting. A Re-examination*. London: Health Visitors Association and United Kingdom Standing Conference on Health Visitor Education.

UKCC (1994) *Standards for the Education & Training of Community Specialist Practitioners*. London: UKCC.

Weinberger, M., Cohen, S. and Mazzuca, S.A. (1984) The Role of Physicians' Knowledge and Attitudes in Effective Diabetes Management. *Social Science and Medicine*, 19, 965–9.

WHO (World Health Organisation) (1984) *Health Promotion: A Discussion Document on the Concepts and Principles*. Copenhagen.

Index